Stumbling Upon the Extraordinary

by

Bill Drover

DORRANCE PUBLISHING CO., INC.
PITTSBURGH, PENNSYLVANIA 15222

ISBN: 978-1-4349-0711-0
Printed in the United States of America

First Printing

For more information or to order additional books, please contact:
Dorrance Publishing Co., Inc.
701 Smithfield Street
Pittsburgh, Pennsylvania 15222
U.S.A.
1-800-788-7654
www.dorrancebookstore.com

To Jeannie

My beginning, middle, and end.

My father says that almost the whole world is asleep. Everybody you know.
Everybody you see. Everybody you talk to. He says that only a few people are awake,
and they live in a state of constant total amazement.
—Patricia, *Joe vs. the Volcano*

Prologue

This is the story of an ordinary guy with ordinary dreams. Growing up, he had simple and common goals: to go to a great college; to meet the girl of his dreams; to get married and have a family; to climb the ranks of corporate America; to buy a big house with a white picket fence…and to live happily ever after.

For anyone who has his or her whole life planned by the age of eighteen, there are many unexpected twists and turns. Throughout his life, he continued to be amazed that what he was seeking was rare, almost freakish.

Along the way, he met many truly remarkable people who caused him to question his aspirations and priorities, to see the world and its inhabitants in a much different light, and to find his true calling.

What follows are thoughts from a man in a constant state of amazement. The special moments are few, but important. They are in no particular order, but that is how life deals them. We don't know when they are coming, no matter what plans we make. But in the end, our time is defined by these precious few, life-shaping events. They give us opportunities to learn, but they must be capitalized upon, for we do not know when they will return.

Introduction

So what the hell does a finance yuppie from Boston know about writing? Truth be told, not much. Math and history were most definitely my favorite subjects. But I know a good amount about relationships, I am a fairly interesting conversationalist, and I feel strongly that many others may benefit from hearing about some of the challenges I have endured.

As my favorite writer, Stephen King, wrote in his book *On Writing,* "Writing isn't about making money, getting famous, getting dates, getting laid, or making friends. In the end, it's about enriching the lives of those who will read your work, and enriching your own life, as well."

I write because, more often than not, personal interactions are limited in time and content, developing not much beyond an initial, "How's it going?" For reasons too numerous to mention, we all take the short road and fire back one of many canned responses:

"Great, how about you?"

"Not bad, can't complain."

There is so much left unsaid, a bottleneck of dialogue that remains trapped, even with those closest to us.

Case in point: my son Nicholas. With a few exceptions, the majority of his immediate family sees him only a handful of times per year. When they do, their interactions with him are brief, for he often chooses to stay in his room, coming down only when called to join others or to seek help with his basic needs—food and bathroom.

Every now and again he will sit on the couch for a few minutes or stay in his chair for a precious moment or two during Thanksgiving dinner, but the sensory overload of sights, sounds, smells, and emotions often are too much for him: the constant chatter from family and friends, all at different pitches and tones; the myriad of smells emanating from the kitchen; family members who have not been part of his routine approaching him, looking for high-fives and hugs. In such moments, Nick characteristically places his index fingers on his ears.

"Too loud?" someone will typically ask.

No, it's too much, and he takes flight into solitude.

So the evaluation from his family is superficial at best. "Nick looks great," they say. "He's always smiling and looks so happy. You guys are doing a great job with him."

Then the inevitable: "How's his progress? Do you think he will ever speak?"

Considering we have spent thousands of hours on his development, including following reams of suggestions and strategies from his Dream Team of educators, where can we begin to answer that question, when most people in the room don't even know what autism is? For that matter, neither do we, not exactly. We know what his challenges are, at least those we can see, but beyond that, it's a crapshoot.

So I write to free up the bottleneck. I don't want to spend hours with our family and friends lamenting our woes; that isn't how my wife, Jeannie, and I approach our challenges. We give each other time to vent, but we focus the majority of our energy on moving forward. Writing helps me unload—and if an accidental consequence is that some day those who care about Nick and us take the time to read about what's really going on, then that's fine as well. I have learned so much about myself over the past four years—the post-diagnosis era—and I believe there are lessons for all of us, if we just take the time to learn.

So here it is: more of a journal than a novel, musings more than story. Like in all of my favorite stories, there is laughter, there are tears, but most of all, there is hope. The ending has yet to be written.

Chapter One

The black limo passed by several times before pulling into our driveway. Two-hundred-year-old farmhouses on equally old roads don't always show up on GPS.

The driver peeked in. His would-be passenger flashed the floodlights, signaling this was the right place. It was a reasonable assumption that he would be the only one on this dark street with a five a.m. pick-up.

As the car turned around in the circular driveway, carefully layered pavers provided plenty of space to point toward the destination: the airport, for another business trip.

I double-checked my belongings: pockets full of tech toys ensuring no lapse in client contact. Even though the out-of-office assistant was turned on, clients would expect a return call. The crackberry provided twenty-four-hour, up-to-the-second access to email; the newest technology even allowed attachments to be opened! I had my cell phone with my work phone number call-forwarded and caller id for over one hundred of my clients. It had download capability for music and movies—perfect for the business traveler. I had my access badge for the office, just in case I needed to stop by after the day's journey, which would end long past bath and story time. My MP3 player was with me, mostly for the plane ride, but also for the likely event that I would be spending hours upon hours in the airport terminal, waiting for the next flight home. I felt like a modern-day cowboy loading his belt for another battle.

Before setting off, I checked one last time on the angels sleeping above. Boy did they look cute—and were they quiet!—when they were sleeping. Both boys were side-sleepers. Their profiles hadn't changed since they lay nose-to-nose in the noisy slumber of the neo-natal intensive care unit.

My wife awoke with me, as she always did no matter the hour, to say "Goodbye," "Good luck," and most importantly, "I love you."

As we headed toward the airport, everything seemed in order. Business trips were a good time to take stock. I ran through the list: great job—senior account manager for a Fortune 500 company; a tenured client base that gave rave recommendations on client-satisfaction surveys and, most importantly, kept their business where it belonged; a fantastic compensation and benefits package; great financial security. As long as I kept up this frenetic pace for the next twenty years, retirement would be a breeze. One year of college was already saved up for each of the four-year-old twins, and we had a half-million in retirement savings—and growing. Not bad for a forty-year-old.

My health had never been better. I finally learned how to eat right: yogurt with almonds gave me a little more energy than a Three Musketeers bar and a Coke. Add in a gym membership, and I was in the best shape of my life. *Men's Health* was good reading on the plane.

Toys: a black Mercedes in the left side of the garage. On office days, it made the three-hour commute a little more enjoyable. The family vehicle was a white minivan—oh wait, no friggin' way! Jeannie drove a metallic gray Volvo SUV.

House: we had waited nearly ten years to find our dream house. Our family of four squeezed into a twelve-room, five-thousand-square-foot antique colonial farmhouse. We had spent the last eight years restoring it, room by room, wavy glass window by wavy glass window—fifty-six in all. In the family room, Barry and Elliot's top-of-the-line sectional faced a sixty-one-inch Samsung. Two acres in the back yard were just waiting for a pool, and we even had enough space for a baseball field. The first few years, I enjoyed cutting the grass myself. But the new life meant much less time at home, so paying one hundred bucks a week to keep the yard nice was a necessary evil.

Okay, was that it for the inventory? *I guess so*, I thought, and I began to nod off. The limo proceeded through the darkened, empty streets of Southern New Hampshire. In the next ten minutes, we would leave the calm complacency of quiet, unlit roads for the hustle and bustle of Route 93 South, the fast lane. Everyone headed as quickly as they could toward somewhere they didn't really want to be.

But something was missing—always missing. What it could be? The midlife crisis? Possibly a tattoo or body piercing would do the trick. How about a weekend at Foxwoods, pissing away a week's salary and catching a bad boxing match? Did I need a Bulgari watch or a Ferragamo tie? I thought not. Most people who judged this book by the cover thought I needed what most middle-aged men in my shoes needed. How accurate was that thought?

My wife and I had spent the last twenty years together. For both of us, this meant more than half our lives. Was it getting old? I began to reflect on how it all had pieced together.

It was the middle of a Triple H summer in the suburbs of Boston, 1986. Lots going on for a twenty-year-old in those parts.

First, and most importantly, the sports scene was never better. The Celtics and Lakers were gearing up for another showdown—Magic vs. Bird. Walton might make the difference this year, we thought, but would his ankles allow him to keep up with Jabbar? Cooper could put Larry in a straight jacket, and The Hick from French Lick still could put up a triple-double and hit the last shot.

The annual ritual of the Impossible Dream, revisited, was playing on Yawkey Way. The young gun from Texas and his lefty counterpart made a great 1:2 combination in the rotation. Oil Can would give you five or six solid innings before falling apart, and The Chicken Man could double off The Monster at will. If only McNamara would watch infield practice and notice that Billy B couldn't bend over to tie his shoes. Oh, well.

The Big Bad Bs were going to the Cup this year. If they only could get past those damn Oilers and that blonde sissy-mary of a hockey player.

The Pats were usually a joke, their less-than-stellar squad filling up the police blotter instead of the metal benches at tired Sullivan Stadium. But they surprised everyone with a trip to the Super Bowl the year before. If I saw The Fridge doing the Superbowl Shuffle one more time, I was going to hurl something at the TV.

Any fan in a major sports city would trade their left nut for four trips to the league championships.

I was cleaning out the basement of my mother's house, listening to AC/DC and planning a night of pounding beers with my other single, broken-hearted, used-and-abused-by-teenage-girls buddies. For some reason, we always allowed ourselves to be manipulated by a group of girls from Eastie. This typically resulted into runs to The Packie, followed by drunken singing on the CB. That's right, the CB: fully equipped with the four-foot-long magnetic antenna, which clung to the roof of any vehicle, but had to be removed if you ever had enough cash for a carwash. It's difficult to believe there actually was a world before cell phones.

The phone rang. I wiped the sweat from my brow and ran up two flights of stairs. It was my sister Karen, calling from work. I wondered what the hell she wanted at this time of the day.

"There's someone here I want you to talk to," she said.

I had no idea where this was coming from. Karen worked in a clothing store, and they occasionally hired hotties to help attract dudes into the store who might need a last-minute Mother's Day present. So it might have been a setup with one of them.

My suspicion turned out to be half-accurate—Jeannie had the look but not the attitude. She was a former employee of Karen's, and my sister had corralled her, shown her some ridiculous prom pictures of this idiot in a white tux with blue-ruffled vest, and professed that she and I would be good together.

"Her name is Jeannie, and I think you would like her."

"Okay, put her on."

We talked for a few minutes, nothing special, and agreed to go out that weekend for dinner. From the tone of our voices, neither of us seemed terribly excited. We both wanted to humor Karen.

When the night of the date came, I realized I had not asked for directions. I called my future best man, a best friend then, who had a photographic memory of all roads in New England. After he provided the directions, I told him I had a date.

"Tonight?" he asked. "Need I remind you this is the first round of hoop playoffs, and we need you? Who is this girl, anyway?"

I had completely forgotten about the game. The decision was an easy one. At this point in my life, choosing whether to play hoops with other sorry-assed losers or go on a blind date was a no-brainer.

"Hi, is Jean home?"

"This is Jean," the obviously masculine voice said. Her father's name had to be Gene, too—not a good sign.

"Who is this?" he demanded. An obviously protective, impatient father—strike two. I told him who I was and why I was calling.

"This is Jean," the sweet voice said.

I then quickly lost my macho, dump-this-chick voice and began to feel nervous. I thought to myself: *Me, actually blowing someone else off?* I mean, I did all right with the ladies, but nothing came easy. In high school, I was smart, but not smart enough to be a geek. I played sports, but not well enough to be a jock. I was a goof-off, but not enough to be labeled a troublemaker. I had friends at all the lunch tables and was an honorary member in most of the cliques. You could measure your popularity in high school by the number of your photographs that made it into the yearbook; I think I appeared in five.

Anyway, I then proceeded to explain to my upcoming blind date about "The Game," as my darling wife now refers to it. Within minutes, the sweet voice turned into a raging volcano. She gave it to me good for a solid two minutes.

I could hear her mother in the background. "Jeannie, who are you talking to like that?"

When she finished, I was speechless. We ended the call one hour before the scheduled pick-up. *That's the end of this one,* I thought.

A few days later, I decided to give it another try. When we started chatting, we sounded like a married couple having an argument, not two pre-adults deciding whether they wanted to hook up. When I finally got up the nerve to ask her to give me another chance, she responded with, "Are you sure you don't have another game?"

Words I will never forget for as long as I live.

Two days later, I pulled into the driveway in my cooler-than-cool black Cutlass Supreme—red velour interior, bucket seats, and a V8. The black exterior showed off the spoked rims and half-landau roof. Oh, I miss that car.

I wasn't nervous at all. I did wonder what she looked like. At least she had seen pictures of me—albeit stupid prom pictures. I did know that she was only seventeen, and I was twenty. It never became an issue; I soon would learn that for her seventeen years, she was more mature than most adults were. Add in the fact that, by most accounts, the gender differential is about five years, and we were practically the same age.

I rang the doorbell. As she came down the stairs and approached the door, I thought of what my sister Karen said: "She has a great personality, she is Italian, and I know you will like her." When she opened the door, I was in shock: "Great personality" usually means nice to talk to, but not so much to look at. But Jeannie had beautiful brown eyes, long, curly brown hair, she was thin, and yes, I did like her—instantly. As she walked up the stairs, I noticed a perfect butt, too.

Something must be wrong here, I thought.

At the top of the stairs, a German Shepherd was waiting to sniff me–test number one. Sabre looked half-wolf, his menacing, white teeth gleaming from the solid-black background of his ninety-pound frame. In truth, he appeared a lot meaner than he actually was.

As time went on, this puppy-dog dressed in ferocious clothing—Jeannie's dad also fit this description—would discover that I worked at Kelly's Roast Beef. We would become instant pals with the delivery of beef scraps several times a week. I quickly received his paw-stamped approval to continue my relationship with his princess.

Meeting Jeannie's mother was a breeze, as was meeting Nana, who lived downstairs. No tests there; they both liked me: college boy, nice car, pleasant manners. My hair was a little long, but their little Jeannie would have that taken care of within a week's time. Say goodbye to the sports bars, strip joints, and nightclubs.

At the end of the first date, there was very little nervousness. We had dinner. I pretended to get lost, but didn't try any cheap moves. She was on to me right away, and we joked about the car running out of gas. The goodnight kiss was a good one. We seemed to know what each other was thinking. I gave her my phone number on a napkin and said I hoped to see her again. I knew I would.

When I got home, my mother asked how it went.

"We clicked," I said.

I could tell she wasn't happy about that. She had seen what the last "serious" teenage relationship had done to me, and she thought I was too young to get seriously involved with girls who had no idea what they wanted. She just wanted me to have some fun without looking for my bride or placing an order for a miniature version of myself. But as much as I tried to act the part of the love-em-and-leave-em type, I was a true romantic and always would be so. I must have the relationship gene in my DNA.

The second date was as smooth, comfortable, and incredibly magical as the first one. We picked up right where we had left off, getting along famously. We talked about everything with the ease of two best friends who had known each other forever. It was also obvious that we found each other attractive.

We were an incredible combination. Our first year together flew by, and at that point, it was only a question of time as to when the big day would come.

There was one minor roadblock. For a brief period, Jeannie wasn't sure of things. After all, we had met when she was sixteen—she had told me a minor lie about her age. But within a year's time, we had a joint bank account and talked openly about marriage. Things were happening fast. Jeannie's doubt did not last long, and soon we both were convinced we would spend the rest of our lives together.

Many people say that kids today don't appreciate each other and don't appreciate the incredible amount of work it takes to form a lasting, loving relationship. In this on-demand, drive-thru, I-want-it-now world, many couples do not invest the time it takes to make the most important decision of their lives. Consequently, courting has become almost extinct, a lost art.

For us, from day one, we were like two old souls suspended in time. It could have been 1986 or 1586. Although we had tremendous respect for others, what mattered most was our unselfishness for each other. Later on, this quality would become the cornerstone of our marriage and the basis for overcoming the many challenges we would face.

Early on, the little things we did for each other built the foundation for our life together. For example, never once did it occur to me to beep the horn when picking her up. I always would go inside, say hi to Nana ("No one came to my door today"), chit-chat a while, open the car door for Jeannie (another chance to look at her butt!), and have her home at a reasonable time.

Most importantly, we both believed in the importance of life's finite details. It's an investment like no other.

From the joint bank account, we went on to buy a hope chest. Most people born after 1970 don't even know what one is. Within a few months' time, it was full of linens and things from family and friends. Best investment we ever made: four hundred bucks for a linen chest that returned four times that in gifts for our future.

The final step was the ring.

There was no doubt in my mind about what I had to do before popping the question. I went to her parents' house one night, just like I did some five nights a week. But this time, I had a diamond in my sweatshirt pocket. So it didn't come with a box—what's the big deal? There was no blood on it, and it appraised for twice what I paid.

I waited for Jeannie to make her final powder room check, and then I made my move. Her father was lying on the couch in a deep trance, the remote control lodged in his hand. He was a retired fireman, a Harley rider; definitely a marshmallow inside, but on the outside, rough-and-tumble. In that moment, a big decision concerning his one-and-only daughter, I saw his true colors—not in his words, but in his eyes.

When I showed him the ring and asked for his blessing to marry his little girl, the result was unexpected. Not only did the remote fall from his hand, but he obviously welled up inside, partly out of love for his daughter and partly out of reciprocal respect for an old-fashioned gesture. I was not quite kissing the ring of the Godfather, but you get the picture. Her father gave his blessing, with the condition that a promise be made to take good care of his only daughter—or else.

By the time Jeannie came back, her father, mother, and I did our best to act natural, as if nothing had occurred. It took everything I had inside of me not to ask her right there, in front of her parents.

I waited until the following day. Her father wasn't home, and her mother was downstairs with Nana. When Jeannie arrived, I was waiting for her, my face as white as a ghost. My palms were sweating like never before. Although we had known each other for more than two years, had saved money, purchased a hope chest, and openly discussed marriage, I was incredibly nervous.

Just as I had asked her father's permission, I knew how I would propose to her. Our timeless, traditional relationship would not be compromised by my screwing up this once-in-a-lifetime moment. I asked her to come into the living room. From the look on her face, I could tell she had no idea what was about to happen. She later told me that she thought it was over.

As she sat down, I knelt down on one knee. My shaking hand reached into my jacket, removing the ring. With my last breath before passing out, I asked, "Will you marry me?"

She was in such a state of shock, I had to ask her again. This was not a good sign. But to my surprise, she accepted, and we called in the spies who were listening at the bottom of the stairs.

As we made the wedding plans, our toughest task (to date) lay ahead. We made up our minds that we would buy a house before the wedding. After one month of looking and six months of hell with banks, mortgage companies, and credit agencies, we were homeowners at the tender ages of twenty and twenty-four.

The wedding was traditional. We simply followed the "suggestions" of our mothers, aunts, and every other female relative. We had a Mass in the church Jeannie grew up attending, a honeymoon cruise to the Caribbean, and a weekend of skiing in New Hampshire—a special time in our lives, indeed. But we just wanted to fast-forward to living under the same roof.

We waited until after the wedding to move into the house. As tradition would dictate, Jeannie's mother had come by to fill the refrigerator and make the bed for the first time. Nana gave the newlyweds a red pepper to keep away the Malocchio, the Evil Eye.

When we returned from our honeymoon, we began to go through everything we had bought, like two kids with birthday presents. Since then, every day has been like the first. The one constant remains: We click, always. Well, mostly.

Chapter Two

Sounds great, right? Just like a Disney movie.

So what was the problem? Was this fairy tale ending? Was Prince Charming getting tired of opening the door for Cinderella, paying his mortgage, and saving for college for his 2.3 kids?

No matter how hard I tried to feel fulfilled with this seemingly perfect life, there was no escaping one simple fact: I could not stand to be away from my wife. It had been that way since day one, and time together just made me love her more and more. There were times I went away for several days on business, playing golf, drinking top-shelf liquor, smoking imported cigars with the other masters of the universe, scheduling the next forty years of our lives in our Blackberries. At the time it seemed like heaven, but at the end of the day—I have grown to hate that corporate cliché—it seemed empty and unsatisfying.

I was a freak.

I had it all, and all I wanted was to spend every minute of my day with my wife and my boys. To me, a bad, rainy day at home doing laundry in my pajamas was better than a seventy-degree day on the golf course. Shoveling dog shit in the yard while the boys played on the swing set gave me more joy than two-day conferences at five-star resorts. Knowing which Wiggle plays the keyboard was more important than memorizing the bio of the new CEO of my most important client.

Even more amazing is that my wife felt the same way. Jeannie had an equally amazing "freak list" of things she would rather do, things that made her happy and that would seem strange to most individuals, never mind couples.

We had met in the most unlikely of circumstances, but our fate was quickly determined over twenty years ago. Maybe fairy tales did come true.

Chapter Three

Once the wedding was behind us, Jeannie and I were anxious about the next phase in our lives. Now came the easy part, right? Nature's simple miracle.

Besides, making a baby should be fun.

Within a year, we decided it was time to grow the family.

Simple enough; just follow the leader. Over the past few years, one by one, our circle of friends checked off each phase in sequential order: engagement, marriage, and then children. Each monthly cycle, we painfully listened to their incredible predictions such as, "I think we will wait until April to get pregnant so we can have the baby in the winter. Then we'll wait thirteen months after the first one is born and have another."

They might as well have ordered up hair and eye color, too. The crazy thing was that, more often than not, it worked out that way.

After the first few months, we began to wonder how long it might take. If Jeannie were still seventeen and we weren't married, this would happen with a wink and a smile. By the time we started tracking the ovulation window, measuring optimum body temperature, and had the first of many exams, it became apparent that nature's most basic function would not happen so easily.

The weeks turned into months, and the months into years. After many heartfelt discussions, we considered that nature would need some intervention. Adoption was also a possibility. Disappointment and sadness gave way to hope.

We both came from the average, American-sized family: three children. Jeannie's mother had her first at the tender age of nineteen, one year into her marriage. The perfect plan.

My parents had the first of three, coincidentally, the same year as their marriage. To this day, I still laugh my ass off every time I call my sister Karen "Love Child".

However, all either family could muster for advice was: "Keep trying; you'll be fine." If they only knew the extent of our efforts.

Most fathers prefer not to hear what their son-in-law is doing to impregnate his daughter. If he knew that much of the work was done in a doctor's office, and that the launch of the mighty swim was done with both doctor and nurse present, that might be more than he could handle.

Our collective strength was never tested more than in our efforts to bring new life into the world. As always, the unselfishness we shared guided us through. Jeannie was amazed at how I handled my end of the agreement, which often included midday sessions with airbrushed women and a plastic cup. I was convinced that my role in the process was minimal compared to what my wife went through. Besides the endless poking, prodding, manipulating, and influencing of her beautiful body, I was more concerned about her mind. What must it feel like to be a female of any species and not be able to complete nature's plan? Although I knew it was not her fault, I could not convince Jeannie that this part was out of our control. A man can never understand fully how this must make a woman feel. So I did my best to be supportive, which often meant keeping my mouth shut.

There were times when I felt helpless. Although we could talk about anything, I was often at a loss for words when the "monthly visit" would crush our hopes yet again. I was as supportive as a man could be, but how can any man relate to a woman whose most basic function has been taken away from her? How would any man feel if it was his equipment that didn't work? If a doctor told him that at age twenty-five, he had the reproductive system of a forty-year-old? The day Jeannie's doctor said that to her, it took all I had to stop me from jumping over the examining table and stabbing him with the scapula. It was the same feeling I would experience many years later, when a young resident would tell me my mother would "expire" within a few months, after her tumor was only partially removed.

There are many times in life when words just complicate matters, offer no explanation, and just muddy the waters. During our decade-long baby quest, there were many such moments.

And the roller coaster ride continued. There were times when it slowed down due to overload. These breaks were necessary to maintain sanity. The select few confidants involved in the inner sanctum, including both mothers, agreed this was a good idea and said, "It's going to happen now that you aren't so focused on it."

If they only knew how powerful "it" was, how all consuming "it" could be, and how this couple battled "it" so ferociously there appeared no end in sight. There were some bright spots, some hopeful moments. But those hopes soon were dashed, and the consequences devastated us like a tornado ripping through a trailer park. We would rebuild, but it would take time. Each time "it" chipped away at the mountain of hope, which was slowly melting like a ski slope in the spring. Jeannie became afraid to think positively, the degree of burns intensifying with each successive crash.

Although individually our strengths diminished, our union grew stronger. The theme of our partnership was and is a simple one: communication. Long conversations, short conversations, and often one-way conversations were the frequent catharsis, an enema to rid the mind, body, and soul of negativity and find additional strength to try again. It was a pattern that would continue throughout our lives. At the time, this challenge seemed to be the highest mountain we would climb. We would be proven wrong. Mount Kilimanjaro would come later.

Chapter Four

At long last, the efforts to build our family began to come together. It started out as a cold, rainy day, the beginning of a long trip far away, never to return. A new home awaited.

She was born in August, a Leo, to a loving mother and father who were victims of a system of economic imprisonment and slavery. There were still parts of the world left behind the social modernization age, still commoditizing life, assigning a price. One after the other, the children were born and sold off. Our little girl had precious few memories of playing with her brothers and sisters. She had been inseparable from her mother. But before long, she was on a plane, off to a far-off destination, waiting to meet her new life and her new family.

Almost a year later, he was born during an unusually cold November in a small New England town. The house was full of siblings, and it became apparent there was not enough room for another hungry mouth. He, too, would be sold to the highest bidder.

They took very different paths, but ended up together in a loving home. For the rest of their lives they would eat, sleep, and play together as brother and sister. Neither cared that their origins were elsewhere. The home where their new family now cared for them was full of love and happiness. Although their parents were not always around, every need was met.

Her journey to this happy place was not a smooth one. When we took her in, we had our doubts. When she was first "purchased," we felt confident she would fill the void missing in our lives. She was worth the money, and we looked forward to getting some return on our investment. A smile, a laugh— any sign to show us that she wanted to be with us. But after the first night, there was a change of heart. Our lost little girl was missing home and was inconsolable all night long. Nothing would soothe her. After much debate and pulling of our heartstrings, we decided to send her home. Maybe adoption was not the answer.

What followed was days of agony. Our hearts and minds were full of conflicting emotions and wonder. Had we done the right thing?

We decided to give it another try. Hopeful that our baby girl had not been sold to another family, we contacted the agency and happily discovered she was still available. Although the next few weeks were filled with nights of weeping and mourning for her lost family, similar to her first night, our young girl soon learned she was loved and this home would be her future.

Our little boy took a different road. His "purchase" was much smoother, and he quickly acclimated himself to his new surroundings. Unlike our girl, who was alone at first, he was quite happy to discover he had a sibling to keep him company when his parents were not around.

They have been through a lot together. As brother and sister, they have witnessed each other's illnesses and prayed for recovery. They each have run away, seeking a better place—or maybe just some attention—only to return to a swift kick in the ass and, eventually, forgiveness.

Each has his or her own unique habits. Our young girl prefers to wander away and roll in any shit she can find, the smellier, the better—preferably big piles of horse shit. She then pretends to shiver when facing her punishment: a long soak in the tub.

Our young boy also loves shit. However, he prefers to chomp on it. His favorite is semi-frozen poopsicles. Although each meal usually is followed by scolding, he cannot resist this delicacy.

Our girl, we call her Patches, loves to sleep. She has been spotted sleeping upside-down, right-side-up, and wrong-side-down. It never has been caught on camera, but we know she can sleep standing up. She also snores like a chainsaw, often with her eyes open, eyeballs rolling around, as we wait for the pea soup to projectile out. Lenora the Snora will appear at any time.

She has been dragged across the bedroom floor, snoozing away, stuck in the closet, and has not lost a beat. On average, she pulls in twenty hours per day. The Queen arises to eat and go to the bathroom, though often not for the latter. She has on occasion let loose in her bed and remained asleep as if nothing has occurred. She will awake in complete denial and blame her brother for the whizzing.

In her early days, she enjoyed escaping from any place, anywhere. She took particular satisfaction in enticing me to chase her around the neighborhood early in the morning—usually while I was still in my pajamas. This was especially fun in the winter, when she could watch me freeze my ass off and grow angrier each minute.

Her favorite meals include leather shoes, ski boots, wedding videos, plaster, and the bottom of any door keeping her locked up. Her love of sports includes hang-gliding. During one hot summer day, a routine escape turned into an adventure when she took off into her neighbor's yard and unknowingly launched herself across a twenty-foot ditch where a retaining wall was under construction. Her crash-landing resulted in an hour-long process to remove four layers of dirt from her teeth.

The boy in our story, Buster, is not as eccentric. If the dog shows handed a ribbon to the largest of breed, you would need three champion beagles to match his sixty pounds. His healthy frame consists of much more than digested dog poop; he will eat just about anything. His favorites include fruits, vegetables, and pig ears. He also has been spotted eating dog food.

Buster also loves to sleep, often in many different places, often during the same night. He will go from the bed to the floor, back to the bed, and back to the floor. While on the bed, he alternates between the full-sprawl horizontal, forcing any other creature with him on the bed to the outer reaches of the mattress, to the under–the-covers horizontal, leaving his masters with a few measly inches of blankets.

He also enjoys quiet rides in the car, glancing out the window, his head snug and close to the driver. He waits for the appropriate time to break the calm and peaceful silence and *woofs* at a blowing leaf or a blade of grass swaying in the wind. This shrilling screech is skillfully positioned directly into the ear of one of his loving parents, prompting them to shit themselves.

Chapter Five

Mature for our ages, but still dreaming of the classic American family, we pressed on. In the beginning, the jokes abounded and actually provided support and encouragement:

"Practice makes perfect."

"This is hard work!"

They got old quickly.

We could not understand why. Had we done something wrong in our lives for which we were being punished? Was it because we were lucky enough to meet each other and build a fairy-tale romance that comes once in a century? Had we filled up our quota from the great-and-powerful being that dishes out happiness?

We were prepared to do whatever it took to have children. We just had no idea what that would entail. The good news was we were living in an area of the country, of the world for that matter, where leading-edge medicine was prevalent. The clinics in and around the Boston area were renowned for their advances in the field of infert…infratil…the inability to make a friggin' baby.

Everyone knows about the Dana Farber and their incredible work with cancer patients. Their relationship with the Jimmy Fund transcends sports and is a topic of conversation during every visit to Fenway. Later on in my life, I would get to know their work intimately.

In the same neighborhood, nestled along Brookline Avenue, just north of Fenway, is the society no one wants to mention. When we walked into a fertility center for the first time, we were amazed at how many others are being tortured through the same methods that we were. Faces sullen, heads down—very few spoke, but no one needed to. The eyes and body language said it all: beaten up, worn down, holding on to a small bit of hope, embarrassed at their inability to perform nature's most basic function.

So what is done to facilitate the simplest process on earth? The possibilities are endless. Once we hit this level, we were in the big leagues. We were well beyond tracking body temperature, putting a pillow in the right place for positioning, or wearing boxer shorts to keep the fish active. We had graduated to a myriad of drugs designed to optimize a woman's body for conception.

The men whose fish couldn't make the swim headed over to the Sperm Bank Drive Thru. They had to check their egos at the door; they couldn't get in if they held on to it too closely. From that point forward, it was no longer about them.

Of course, preparing the miracle drugs was nothing short of getting a degree in pharmacology. At one point, I almost "borrowed" a lab coat from one of the clinics to bring some humor to the situation. I pictured me and Jeannie, drunk (from mental exhaustion—no parts liquor in this concoction), mixing the potions in those fat-bottomed glass bottles like the ones from eleventh-grade chemistry class. I chickened out, settling for referring to Jeannie as Beaker, my favorite Muppet.

The monthly ritual included endless blood tests to determine the magic window of opportunity, mixing these magic potions, injecting them, and then heading back to the clinic for the critical insertion. The miracle moment would now, hopefully, happen in a doctor's office. Not very romantic, but the result was what mattered. Keeping perspective was paramount. But even with the innovative medicine, the days, months, and years continued to crawl by. Many times we were on the verge of giving up, of resigning ourselves to the fact that our family would be limited to the furry little ones and each other.

Infertility is taboo, especially when it comes to family. We soon found out that it wasn't just our parents who couldn't understand what impact it could have on individuals and on relationships, even magical ones such as ours. Siblings, with their own children in tow, seemed oblivious. Best friends offered little support or consolation. Jeannie and I had each other, they must have reasoned, a special relationship that could overcome anything. I'm sure they thought, "They'll work it out." It was another theme that would continue throughout life's bumpy road.

But weren't we handed this relationship as a special gift, a perfect match that could overcome any obstacle? And weren't we two people who were built the same way, with the same raw materials that brought out the best in each other by being unselfish, caring, and putting first the needs of the other? Sounds like a tale from Greek mythology: created as a model of ideal love, a reward typically reserved for the Gods. But you cannot procreate: So it shall be written.

We soon became uncle and aunt, godfather and godmother many times over. The joy of being part of other growing families was bittersweet: We held babies in our arms, but we knew we may never experience that with one of our own. We vicariously dreamed about baby pictures, the first crawl, first words, and having spit-up on our shoulders.

One day we found ourselves in a place we had visited many times: a holding pattern. We had done our part. Now it was time to watch the calendar and wait for the fertility gods to render their decision. We had programmed ourselves through reverse psychology not to get our hopes up; the call from the doctor's office would yield the same results it always did, and if we had chosen to utter, or even think about the "P word", we would crash and burn.

Jeannie was sitting in the rocking chair when the phone rang. As I stood beside her, I could not help but perk up, mustering one last drop of wishful thinking. As I watched her body language, my heart sank again.

I remembered the day some fourteen years ago when I held her engagement ring in my hand and prepared to get down on one knee. The same lightlessness passed through my body, and I floated toward her. Was this another cruel, torturous test, or was she actually smiling? I could not hear anything coming from the caller, but what I heard from Jeannie's beautiful mouth will remain with me forever:

"And you are sure it's multiples?"

Chapter Six

Before we knew it, Jeannie was horizontal under a myriad of beeping machines and strobe lights, jelly on her belly. The great thing about having twins was that we had an ultrasound every month. At first it was cool to carry them around. The glossy black-and-white photos came in strips, like those you could get in a two-dollar mini photo machine at the bowling alley.

When we saw our first view of the twins, I stared at the pictures long and hard, trying to find their tiny bodies within the blackness of the mini X-rays. If I looked closely enough, I could make out the rough outline of a curled-up little critter—or two! It was like trying to spot a car from thirty thousand feet up in a streaming jetliner: just a bunch of ants crawling around.

"Yeah, I think I see a head. How come there's only one?" *Oh shit, here we go again.* We'd already lost one of the twins. We'd been trying for four thousand goddamn days, two hundred monthly cycles, and I don't want to count how many broken promises (three to be exact). Just when we had programmed ourselves not to believe any more, we had been fooled again. I wasn't so sure we could take it this time around.

"The other one is not visible because one of your boys is sitting on his brother's head," the doctor explained.

"Boys? Those are *my boys* in there?" I said. *Holy shit!* I was going to be a dad.

During those first few months, we were still in disbelief. We had experienced disappointment after disappointment and were waiting for the roof to cave in yet again. As was the case with virtually every cycle during the past decade, the moments passed excruciatingly slowly. *So what the hell do I do now?* I thought. *I guess I'll go back to worrying.* I love reverse psychology. If I believe long and hard enough that it never will happen, then it will.

There was a time in my life when those thoughts were reserved for The Boys of Summer. In Beantown, the ritual every fall, just before the leaf-peepers would head into town, was to lament the Curse of the Bambino. Little did I know, not only would the curse be reversed—twice—during the first few years of my boys' lives, but my life would tip in the direction of a non-hysterical reaction: "Hey, that's great. I am glad they finally won it." Once I held those miracles in my arms, I officially was excommunicated from the I-can-die-now-that-they-have-won-a-World-Series club. I guess it just wasn't that important after all. Well, maybe a little.

Once we had passed the "probationary period" of three months, the news was out. I loved to take the ultrasound pictures to work with me.

"Hey, take a look at my little ones."

"Nice picture. Is she giving you the finger?"

"No, it's a *he*, asshole. Can't you tell? And *he* is sitting on *his* brother's head."

"Oh, you've got two in there? Good luck, man. With two boys, they'll be at each other all the time. I'm sure they will be sitting on each other's heads quite often, running around playing ball, and doing everything together."

Hey, that sounded incredible. I couldn't wait.

If I were showing the pictures to a woman, she would say, "Twins? I always wanted to have twins."

But as the months rolled by and the double-decker started to wreak havoc on my wife's beautiful body, I wasn't so sure any woman would want to give birth to twins.

The pregnancy was very different from anything else we had experienced. During the engagement, we were in control of our destiny. We could decide to save money, buy a hope chest and a house, have impact on our future. But during the pregnancy, two Type A personalities, neither of whom had lived life moment-to-moment, were sent back in time to a place where we hoped we would never return. As Dr. Seuss described in *Oh, the Places You'll Go!*, it was:

A most useless place. The Waiting Place...for people just waiting.
Waiting for the phone to ring, or the snow to snow
Waiting around for a Yes or No.

This time we weren't waiting for magic to happen. This time we were waiting for hell to consume us, because if it happened again, if we lost them, that's what the rest of our lives would have felt like.

But the months went by, and the pendulum began to swing toward excitement. As we turned into the homestretch, Jeannie prepared to drag her battered body into the doctor's office for an "observation." The upcoming doctor's appointment was right around her birthday, smack in the middle of the hazy, hot, and humid days of August.

With her license about to expire, Jeannie headed off to the Registry of Motor Vehicles with my dad in tow, since I was out of town on business for the day. Men could care less about the photo they will carry in their wallet for the next four years. If anything, they might hope it looks good enough to hang on the wall in the post office. Women, of course, approach this event quite differently.

Jeannie and my dad walked into the registry, soaked in sweat. Thirty-two weeks pregnant with twins, limbs swollen and bloated, and her beautifully curly hair out of control (think Frieda in Peanuts), she took her license photograph.

Meanwhile, I was getting paid way too much money to talk to someone I barely knew in an air-conditioned conference room. What's wrong with such a picture? And back at the registry, none of the assholes waiting their turn gave up their seat for Jeannie. I'm just glad I wasn't there, as I probably would have gotten arrested for throwing someone on the floor.

Fortunately, I arrived home from the business trip in time to join Jeannie for her doctor's appointment. Her physician had grown increasingly concerned about her fluid buildup and wanted to avoid toxemia. As we sat in the post-examination room, the nurse came in and said something I could barely hear. I saw her lips move, heard the faint sounds come out of her mouth, but could not make out the meaning. It was the same feeling I had after I had proposed to Jeannie, when I heard my mom's doctor announce stage-four ovarian cancer, and when I heard Jeannie say, "And you're sure it's multiples?"

"You are not going home," the nurse explained.

Huh?

"You are having the babies this weekend, probably within the next few days. Go home and pack a bag, Bill."

Huh?

The next thing I knew, I was on the way back home, and Jeannie was in an ambulance on her way to a hospital with a level-three NICU. Over the next forty-eight hours, a medical SWAT team swooped in and out of Jeannie's room providing medicine for her to fight the toxemia and medicine for the boys to build their lungs. "We want them breathing on their own right away," the doctors explained.

Yeah, no shit. So do I.

Jeannie had a monitor on her belly tracking every movement, every bodily function—hers and the boys'. It even tracked the temperature on the moon. The thing beeped every three seconds. Good thing I packed extra underwear, because I must have soiled myself a dozen times—and the delivery hadn't even started yet.

Afterward a doctor walked in, rubbed his beard, and proceeded to give us the details for the birth certificate. One baby was four-and-a-half pounds, and the other was about three-and-a-half, give or take a few ounces. They both were about seventeen inches long.

I felt like asking him, "Do you have names picked out?"

Over the past decade, through the long and arduous task of getting to this point, we had become accustomed to scheduled events. The magic of pregnancy vanished long ago with the tracking of body temperature, counting of days in the cycle, and mixing of magical potions. Getting us pregnant was akin to Luke Skywalker connecting on the one-in-a-million laser shot that detonated the Death Star.

So we looked at our doctor with eyes, mouths, and hearts wide open.

"Tonight at six-thirty. See you then."

"Okay. I guess it's a date," Jeannie said.

"Anything else we need to know?"

"Yeah."

The next, most important question for me was on its way. The doctor looked up from his clipboard, scanned me, seemingly sizing up my ability to deal with what was next in this process, and asked, "Can you handle the epidural? Because most husbands pass out at the sight of the needle. We've got enough to do here without having to help you off the floor."

Chapter Seven

I guess I couldn't handle the big needle.

Left outside the prep room, I paced the empty hallway. One of the wall-mounted TVs was on in a vacant room. Inside, the perfectly made bed lay empty; bedpans hid underneath; the adjustable tray waited for its next meal; a plain box of tissues, full, sat on the nightstand.

I peeked in the room and glanced at the screen. I knew that sound—sports! As if someone were watching over me, it wasn't "Masterpiece Theatre" or even QVC. Saturday night, August 25, 2001—it was the Little League World Series. Of course, there was no way our team of eleven- and twelve-year-olds could compete with the teams from across our borders with the phony birth certificates. On that night, our boys from Apopka, Florida had just won the United States Championship. Their reward: the unfair challenge of taking on the young men from Tokyo in the next day's championship game.

Sports! Can you believe it? What else did the mighty poker dealer have in store for me? Was this a theme? Oh, I love themes. How about a World Series Championship? Two? No way. Throw in three Super Bowl Rings and an NBA title! Oh, come on. Let's not get carried away. First they needed to get my miracles out of my wife's body before all three of them drown in toxic fluid. Then we could visit sports heaven.

Hello, time to focus! They called me in to the delivery/operating/excavation room, where the miracles were about to make their appearance. This room was nothing like the chocolate room in Wonka's factory; it was bland, but had warm colors on the walls. The only common thread: magic.

There are a lot of people in here, I thought.

The doctor quickly guided me bedside, next to my wife. At Jeannie's mid-point, there was a curtain dividing the giver and the receivers. Four anesthesiologists—okay, maybe three—had put her into a semi-conscious state, while the pitcher, first baseman, shortstop, and third baseman assumed their positions, my wife at home plate. They all were awaiting the delivery.

The suction team was standing by, like the grounds crew waiting to sprint onto the field during a rain delay. They were equipped with a giant vacuum hose, like the ones that cost seventy-five cents for two minutes at the exit of the carwash—the ones that can suck the watch off your wrist.

What the hell do they need that for? I didn't want to know.

During the process, there were moments when I thought I, too, was high on ether, as I could have sworn I saw one of the doctors jump on Jeannie's belly to force the boys out.

Inside, the boys formed the shape of a *T*: Nick was, in fact, sitting on Joe's head, a scene we wouldn't see repeated until they were almost eight years old.

The baseball analogy quickly turned into the Big Dig, as the excavation seemed to go deeper into the chasms of the hospital, through the basement and into the center of the earth to grab my children. *There must be a hole in my wife!* I thought. *How can she not be feeling this?*

The only time I stood up to get a peek, Joseph was on his way out. Only it wasn't Joseph—it was the Baby Grinch. I did get to hold him for a brief second, but the nurse quickly cleaned him up and put him in the egg cooker, which was sitting curbside to Jeannie's gurney. Three minutes later, his brother Nick arrived, equally gooey, following the same route as his brother. Although not quite aware, Jeannie did manage a quick peek, a huge smile, and then a sigh of relief.

Chapter Eight

After the excavation—eh, birth—the boys lay asleep, two floors above Jeannie's room. They had reservations for two in the incubator suite. Good thing they had twenty-four-hour room service: "We'll need sunglasses for the bright lights that bring us life. We'll need some lotion on our eyes, as this light is way too strong. We are too tired to eat, so please just stick a tube up our noses and into our bellies. Yeah, that's it. Some more milk, please. And where the hell is our mother?"

Once again, we were blessed to be in the epicenter of the medical world. At thirty-two weeks, our miracles were early, but there was an air of confidence mixed with caution from the staff that cared for them: "So far, everything looks great. They are breathing on their own, no machines. No sign of infection, and they have good appetites."

We, on the other hand, were scared shitless. At a combined weight of less than eight pounds, our boys were tiny, and we were back to counting seconds, minutes, and hours. As their lives began, we kicked off parenthood as spectators—sort of. We did get to see them, to touch them, but for the first few days, it was through the rubber-gloved biodome of a home. Already we could see our boys were rare, for sure. We needed them to be medium-well, so the cooker cooked on.

I had spent the last three nights in the hospital with Jeannie. Our first, furry children, Buster and Patches, were in good care with their Papa (my dad) and Nana (Dad's second wife) and their dog, (Uncle) Casey. I guess my dad's dog would be my brother if we drew it on the family tree. Three beagles spending time together: one less thing to worry about.

After sleeping in Jeannie's purple silk pajamas on the makeshift bed in her room ("It's a chair and a bed! Order now and get two for the price of one, and we'll waive shipping!"), I made my way north, headed home for a hot shower, some male clothing and a good night's sleep. Little did I know that as soon as

I had left, Jeannie had been whisked away to not only see, but cuddle her boys for the first time. Although I was not there, through the magic of Sony video and Polaroid instant film, I did get to relive the first physical connection between the love of my life and the new loves in my life. Fortunately for me, there would be many, many similar moments over the next few weeks, months, and years.

At that moment, a turning point happened in our lives. If I think back to high school English, I believe they called it a "denouement." As defined by Wikipedia, a denouement "consists of a series of events that follow the climax of a drama or narrative, and thus serves as the conclusion of the story. Conflicts are resolved, creating normality for the characters and a sense of catharsis, or release of tension and anxiety, for the reader." Yeah, that's it. We had one of those. We experienced closure on the most significant challenge in our life to that point. Although the situation was still quite bizarre, I did feel a sense of normalcy. And as for the tension and anxiety, I'm sure you can draw your own conclusion.

Chapter Nine

After four long days in the level-three NICU of St. Elizabeth's Medical Center, our boys were ready for transport. Boot camp was complete, and they were in good enough shape to ship off to Lawrence General, home of a very competent NICU, thank you very much. It was time for another ambulance ride—woo hoo! Only this time, we had two extra passengers. Joe and Nick were strapped in more robustly than Hannibal Lecter during a visit from Clarise Starling. We headed north and arrived in Lawrence happy and hopeful.

The initial forecast was to keep them until at least week thirty-five, the standard benchmark for preemies to be able to go home. Of course, there was a long list of other milestones they needed to achieve before we could completely call them our own. But in time, each achievement would come. For the moment our days consisted of morning, afternoon, and evening shifts shuffling back and forth from home to hospital.

During the first few weeks, the NICU simultaneously was a minimum-security prison—equipped with ankle bracelets for the boys, like those reserved for fancy white-collar criminals on house arrest—and an institute for higher learning. We had no idea what we were doing, and we learned firsthand from experts (who also happened to be angels). We soon became experts in many fields, including the basics such as feeding and diaper changes. These tasks might sound simple, but with the myriad of wires attached to their tiny bodies, great care and precision was critical. Good thing we were both anal-retentive Type A personalities, good list-makers and planners. As you might have guessed, Jeannie is the only one, however, who can read directions, especially for toy assembly or reading a map. I claim the male gene on that one.

As the weeks went by, we graduated from having no idea what to do to having some sense of how not to let them die of starvation or drown in their own pee. What else was there? *Oh, just wait, my friend,* someone from the future would have said to us. *There is much more in store for you.*

One morning, just like many other work days, I recall sitting in a conference room waiting for another nonsensical meeting to begin. It was eight forty-five on a beautiful September day. Glancing out at the blue sky, I wished I was elsewhere—not sitting in the box seats at Fenway, not in my backyard chasing my dogs around, but in the jam-packed nightclub of a nursery in Lawrence, Massachusetts, with babies crying, parents crying, and machines beeping. I was sure Jeannie was there giving one of the boys a bath or trying to get them to drink four ounces of milk without throwing up.

The date was September 11, 2001, and we all know what happened next. My fellow worker bees crowded into the video conference room and watched the footage play repeatedly, our mouths open, speechless. We were a room full of bullshit artists who could not muster a single word.

An hour later, I arrived at the temporary home for my family. Jeannie and I looked into each other's eyes. No words were necessary. I will not attempt to describe the magnitude of the moment, as what happened on that day affected so many lives other than the three most important ones in my world. All I know is that never in my life have I felt a stronger sense of where I belonged than in that moment.

Chapter Ten

Baby A and Baby B were their names for about three hours. Many times I have been asked why we did not name one of the children after me. My dad was also a William, as was his father.

My answer: "How could I do that?"

"What do you mean?" would be the typical response. "They're your children. You can name them anything you want."

No, sir. No way. Years later, one of my boys might come up to me and say, "Dad, why did you name my brother after you? Do you love him more than me?" Make no mistake: My love and my pride for my boys could fuel the next space shuttle; but my ego could not.

Each day we waited for the green light from the doctor. As he ran through the checklist of milestones, we hoped for boarding passes back to New Hampshire. Finally, we got our wish—sort of. Joseph was ready to come home, but Nick was not.

"Nothing to worry about," the doctor said. "He just needs a few more days with some closer monitoring."

With mixed emotions, we put Joseph in the car seat and headed home. Part of us remained with Nick.

We also realized we were on our own now. Like most parents, we were nervous about becoming the number-one caregivers for our child. Deep down inside, we both knew we could more than handle it. I know Jeannie won't admit it, even to this day, but she has a quiet confidence and a relentless pursuit of excellence. Simultaneously she can get great joy in life's moments while always striving to do better. She won't admit she is a good mother, a good wife, or a good daughter. I could spend the rest of this tale building irrefutable cases that would convict her on all counts of being a superb example of all three, but we'll save that for later. For now, trust me. The Jeannies of the world come once in a lifetime. Lucky for me, I scored one.

The first night with Joseph was special in so many ways. As we walked him upstairs to the waiting nursery, it didn't feel right. It was the same feeling we had when we closed on the house three months before the wedding, and the same reason we left it vacant until we returned home from our honeymoon. I also think it's the same reason the spirits in our two-hundred-year-old colonial, which we now call home, leave us alone.

"Let me hang out on the couch with him for a little while," I said to Jeannie.

As I look back on that first night, there were so many emotions. Part of me wanted to get him acclimated to his new surroundings. The other part of me just wouldn't let him go. So I held him. And I held him...all night and into the morning, with a couple diaper changes and feedings thrown in. I guess I figured the best way to make sure he was okay was to keep him in my arms. There would be plenty of time to teach him about his new world.

Four days later, our family became complete with the addition of Nicky into our funhouse. Over the next four months, life visiting the boys at the NICU was replaced with twenty-four-hour shifts of diaper changes, feedings, laundry, and sneaking in a peanut-butter-and-jelly sandwich. Fortunately, both Jeannie and I usually performed well with structured tasks. After the first few weeks, I could change a diaper and empty the Genie quicker than the pit crew changes a tire at the Indy 500. The inventor of the Diaper Genie should receive the Nobel Prize for innovation—I love that thing!

Chapter Eleven

It was Christmas morning, four months to the day from when the boys entered our lives. I recall waking up and seeing the sun.

"What the hell time is it?" I asked. I leaned over in bed, expecting to see either Buster's balls or Patches's cookie staring me in the face. We definitely should have crate-trained them.

Instead, I saw Jeannie. "Did you get up last night?" we asked simultaneously.

Holy shit. We fell asleep and forgot to feed them, change them, cuddle them, read and sing to them. I couldn't believe we fucked this up so quickly. We didn't deserve to have children! We leapt out of bed and ran over to the crib, terrified of what we might find. They were less than fifteen feet from us, and we let them slip away. As we each grabbed one, our collective memories must have awoken our senses of smell. Jeannie's nose recalled urine, and I smelled poop. They did live! I couldn't believe they were still alive!

We consulted our nighttime log and deduced it had been nearly seven hours since either of them had eaten or had a diaper change. In that moment, we realized many things—most importantly, they were strong little buggers, and they were ours. What we received that morning never showed up on my list to Santa, but we got it anyway: validation that we could do this parenting thing, and a good night's sleep to boot.

Merry Christmas!

Chapter Twelve

As if overnight, the turkey timer popped out on our once-rare preemies, and they quickly turned into what I can best describe as footballs. I'm not talking Nerf or even American footballs. They looked more like the ones used to play rugby: long, pale white, and round in the middle. I mean, they filled in, from head to tippy-toe: their heads, their necks, their midsections, their legs, and their feet. It looked like someone had taken a tank of helium and filled them up. Bouncers from Beantown: no problem getting a job back at the NICU Nightclub. My buddy Eddie nicknamed them Nicky Pockets and Joey Bag of Donuts. Badda Bing, Badda Boom!

We do have lots of video of both boys eating a long list of foods they won't touch now. The evidence might as well be inadmissible to our seven-year-olds who only eat hot dogs, chicken nuggets, and orange goldfish crackers. But once upon a time, they ate everything they could get their hands on—food, that is. Not sure what else they might have consumed while we weren't watching. Hey, I ate my fair share of dirt as a child, and I'm none the worse for wear!

Oh shit, I just sounded like my dad. "I don't need to worry about what I eat," he often would say. "Weight has never been a problem for me." Okay, Dad, but the two ulcers, the stroke, the quadruple bypass—could they be signs of a less-than-healthy interior? But I haven't become my father; I have become *his* father. We truly are the "sandwich generation", caring for our children and our parents at the same time.

As Jeannie and I watched life growing right before our eyes, the opposite was happening in a parallel universe. My mother's cancer had taken a turn for the worse. For the past three-and-a-half years, she had fought as much as she could to maintain her strength, her dignity, and her place in the family she had built. Her 'life in prison' was about to be commuted, replaced by a death sentence. Just as my world was filling up with two more members of the I-can't-get-enough-of-you club, the most important person in the first half of my life was preparing to leave me. It was way too soon. We were just getting to the good stuff. She would not be around to be a part of the next phase in her sons' journeys, journeys for which she had prepared me and that I know she would be proud to witness.

During her short time with the boys, she did manage to get some joy from them. In the end, her immune system had become so weak that holding the boys in her arms required extra precautions. I recall her holding Joseph, surgical mask over her mouth, her once-straight hair that had grown back as a batch of curls. In her eyes, I could see many things: the love, the hope, and the pride that she had sent my way so many times in my life; but also sadness and regret. She wouldn't see our boys shaking their legs at the dinner table. She wouldn't play Scrabble with them or watch them run up and down the hall with their baseball gloves on, pretending to make a game-saving catch. They wouldn't make her laugh hysterically as I had done so many times in her life.

In her final few days, my sisters and I spent as much time with her as possible. She was home; nothing else could be done for her within the white walls of the miracle-makers on Brookline Avenue. No more magic potions to wage war with the enemy inside her. No more knives to remove the parts of her body that had succumbed. No more fighting. It was her time. At just shy of sixty years old, it was much too early.

Each night we would take turns sleeping on the floor by her bed. She had been there for all of us, for every important moment of our lives. There was no way she was going to leave us while she was alone. So as we waited for death to take her, we were visited by another charter member of the Angels on Earth club.

In the Glossary, I have included a list of words I never knew existed. We should add "hospice" to that list. I don't even recall the hospice worker's name; all I can remember is her strength. She was there to comfort us as a family and to prepare us for what was about to come. At the same time, she cared for our mother in ways that a mother cares for her infants. I could not bear to see my hero in a diaper, nor would she want me to see her that way.

On what would be her final night on earth, I had decided to go home and check in with Jeannie and the boys. The 24/7 shift had calmed down somewhat as our six-month-old bags of cement began to settle in to a more regular, insane schedule.

The next morning, I grabbed a cup of coffee from Double Ds and headed back to my mother's apartment. It was shift change, so my sisters could do what I had done the night before: sleep in my own bed, have a decent meal, and temporarily take my focus off the imminent death of my mother. On my way down, I got the call from Karen, the same Karen who had called me some sixteen years before to set me up on a blind date with some Italian girl I had never met. I guess she is the gatekeeper for the most important people in my life.

When I arrived, the ambulance was there. As they brought in the gurney, the empty body bag sat on top. In another ten minutes, it was zipped up, containing the most influential person in my life. She taught me everything: how to love, how to laugh, how to be independent, and how to persevere.

I miss her every day of my life.

Chapter Thirteen

It began innocently enough. During the first year or so, Nick actually seemed to be progressing more quickly than his brother in communication (he babbled, but he gave lots of eye contact), walking, and appetite. Watching him every day, I thought he seemed like the typical kid: always smiling and very interactive with us and with his brother.

Between his second and third year, his development plateaued and then began to regress. The sensory issues began to surface. His feet were an obvious sensory challenge; Nick did not want to put on or keep on his shoes. He constantly walked on his tiptoes. His once-hearty appetite turned into an aversion to foods, sometimes based on texture or shape. To this day, only certain colored jellybeans or Starbursts will enter his mouth. Most of his favorite foods are bland and crunchy: pretzels, goldfish crackers, and Cheerios.

His lack of understanding of social settings and appropriate behavior was also noticeable. We did not expect our toddler to write an Emily Post essay, but it was obvious he did not know how to communicate. If someone presented him with something to eat or drink or asked him if he wanted to read a book, his negative response typically would take the form of the back of his hand—not to the person, but to the object.

Nick began to demonstrate repetitive behaviors. One of his favorite activities was watching videos. The *Baby Einstein* series was—and still is for Nick at age seven—a wonderful way for him to learn many rudimentary concepts such as colors, shapes, and music. While watching videos, Nick would repeat a series of body movements: three steps back, three steps forward, followed by a smack to the TV screen; he obviously was not in control of all his sensory stimulation.

Nick exhibited unusual "play". He was proficient at fifty-piece puzzles at a very early age, but he had trouble playing with the most basic of toys. One Christmas he received a wooden tool bench. Nick had difficulty figuring out which piece was the hammer and how to use it. When we would demonstrate the many "proper" ways to play—sounds awful, doesn't it?—he would rebel, shut us out, and do it his own way.

His gross motor skills such as running, jumping, and balance were strong. However, his fine motor skills—holding an object in his hand like a crayon or a utensil or using his index finger to point or touch—were major challenges and continue to be so.

The most significant and painfully obvious sign of trouble was the blank stare. Eye contact was rare. The insanity of having a healthy, happy, smiling boy whom you could look right through was almost unbearable. His emotions seemed almost robotic.

"Nick, Daddy loves you."

He would give me his chin to connect with mine. Then he would go back to his routine, lining up his toys, completing one of his puzzles. Any break in that routine, if a puzzle piece would be lost or become stuck on the board, would result in an explosion. Nick typically would express his frustration by crying loudly and escaping to his safe place of solitude: He would shut out the world by covering his ears.

If I said, "Daddy loves you" ten times a day, he would repeat the same action each time.

I recall heading off for work, and Nick wouldn't even acknowledge I was leaving. I typically would return twelve hours later, and it was almost as if he didn't realize I was gone. If I went on a business trip for two or three days, I would be met with the same result.

Although Nick did make sounds, as he does today, he did not form any words. His mode of communication consisted of grabbing us by the hand and taking us to what he wanted: the bathroom, the refrigerator, or to the door. When he wanted to be alone, he escorted us out of his space so he could escape to his solitude.

During holidays, relatives who would only see him every few months would note that he seemed so happy, so content: "You two are so lucky to have two healthy boys!" But if they spent more than a few minutes with Nick and watched his twin brother, they would begin to understand that the last statement was not so accurate.

As we approached their third birthday, we knew it was time to get some help. Because the boys were preemies, we qualified for professional assistance through Easter Seals and the Early Intervention Program. We began speech and physical therapy. Early on, the speech sessions were very difficult. Nick's frustration in not being able to communicate often came across very loudly. Unlike many other children on the autism spectrum, Nick did not become physical with any of his providers. He did, however, become physical with himself.

For Nick, his chin has always been the focal point of his sensory system. During his early development years, when he was presented with a task he did not like or the inability to communicate his needs, he would whack his chin with the palm of his hand. The pros called this "organizing", which I never fully grasped, but here's my level of understanding: We all process the inputs we receive from our five senses. When Nick's inputs get clogged up, he needs to re-organize—to clear the blockage. For some, this task might be accomplished by closing their eyes. Others might concentrate on their breathing. Still others might use their own words in an attempt to calm the body. For Nick, and for other children on the spectrum, the inputs and corresponding responses between the nervous system and the brain are broken. His sensory nucleus is his chin. I guess you could call it his reset button.

Our speech therapist also spent time with Joseph. As he was just three minutes older than his brother, Joseph also qualified for individual speech sessions. "Why not?" Jeannie and I agreed. We had been duped during Nick's first few years, and it was now clear he was not "typically developing". Who knew what was lying in wait for Baby A?

After the fifth session with Joseph, we looked into Judy's eyes. She was an angel—another of the many to appear in our average lives. Her business card read "Speech and Language Pathologist". Through her years teaching adolescents how to communicate, Judy had come across many different students with varying needs. When we asked about Joseph's communication skills, she smiled. It was as if she could look into the future and view him as a seven-and-a-half-year-old boy who never stops talking until he falls asleep. He would become a spelling bee runner-up in the second grade, proficient at Scrabble, a lover of Search-a-Words.

She also knew what was wrong with Nick. Ironically, Judy couldn't use words to tell us—a barrier in her profession, but not in her eyes. Once we did some research and figured out what autism was, we knew that she knew. All that was left was the formal diagnosis. During our one and only trip to the neurologist, the MRI confirmed no brain damage. A detailed evaluation also yielded the formal declaration: autism—no known cause, no known cure, and an uncertain future. We had no answers to our questions: *Will he live a normal life? Will he ever speak? Will he be able to take care of himself?* No answers, only questions; not even speculation.

To say we were devastated might be obvious, but not completely accurate. When we got the news that my mother was diagnosed with stage-four ovarian cancer, and later when Jeannie's dad would be diagnosed with ALS, we had a pretty good idea what the future held. When someone tells you, however, that your son has a developmental disorder affecting the functioning of the brain, it gets your attention. When they tell you they are unsure of how it will affect his development, you become frighteningly curious. So where could we go from here? If the world's top specialists could not discover the cause or chart a course for the cure, what the hell were we supposed to do?

Fortunately, or unfortunately, there are others on this planet who have similar challenges, and we soon would be introduced into another underground society. It was similar to our experience with infertility. We were shocked when we saw the numbers of families impacted by this diagnosis, and we again entered into a world we never knew existed, a world of everyday people dealing with not-so-everyday challenges that completely consumed their lives. Thank goodness all the public servants in this magical place had white wings.

I remember our first day at School Administration Unit 28 in Windham, NH. I didn't realize it then, but it's an incredibly challenging assignment for the professionals who work with our special kids every day. As parents, we show up with a myriad of emotions: anger, frustration, confusion, fear, and often blame. For some reason, many parents blame the caregivers for the fate of their children. As caregivers, their job is to eliminate the noise—which is often the family—and focus on the results. To say this requires special skill is a gross understatement.

For the next three years, Jeannie and I were introduced to many strategies (read: no cures) designed to augment the development of our son, to prepare him for the next stage in his life, and to arm us with tools to continue his development at home. When you speak with folks who deal with autism, they never use the C word. Not only does it not exist, but it is counterproductive. There are no special medicines to counteract this disease, no proven protocols to make it go away—only therapies to help deal with its destructive impact on the body and mind.

Jeannie and I quickly would learn we needed to redefine many terms in our life: patience, progress, and most importantly, perspective.

Chapter Fourteen

During Nick's three-year stint at SAU 28, he made great strides. Our biggest challenge was not to compare Nick's progress with Joseph's. As a blooming flower at the local Montessori School, Joseph quickly began to display that he, too, was not typically developing. However, his atypical development was more smile-worthy: Joseph made friends easily; he quickly emerged as a leader in his class.

Joseph was simultaneously a four-year-old boy discovering all the wonders of the world and a young man struggling to understand complex life issues by becoming a caretaker and advocate for his brother. As a sibling of a disabled child—it took us a long time to admit to that—we recognized early on that Joseph would grow up more quickly than he should. The sacrifices he needed to make to accommodate the special needs of his brother, the curious looks that others sent his brother's way, the unanswered questions about why Nick does what he does: they all matured him quickly. So we continued to pay close attention and tried to make sure Joseph experienced life as a four-year-old boy, even though he sometimes acted thirty-four.

To enable Nick to be successful, the first thing I needed to do was to get over myself. My system of measurements, of milestones, and of successes went out the window. I have to admit it was a humbling moment when my son received high marks on his progress report for touching his nose five times without request. This moment was contrary to the first forty years of my life. The bar was always set high, and I spent every ounce of my energy trying to clear it.

At the same time we were adjusting our expectations for Nick, we also were raising them for Joseph. This careful balance required much thought and regulation. Our parental skill set for our toddler twins had many different tools. It was more like having a one-and-a-half-year-old and an eight-year-old. Every parent needs to understand each of their children's potential and adjust his or her expectations accordingly. We certainly had that challenge with our boys.

Chapter Fifteen

"Oh look, twins! What's your name?"

"Joseph."

"And how about you, handsome?"

"That's my brother, Nick; he uses pictures to talk."

For Joseph, the irony of having a playmate, someone to share a room with, share a swing set with, take baths with, but not to have reciprocal play with often could lead to frustration. We were so blessed that Joseph understood and made sacrifices for his brother and the family's well-being. But still, there were moments.

How do you respond to: "Mom, why do you have two boys? I thought you only wanted one?" Or, "Did you want two normal boys like me, or did you want one like me and one like Nick?" And, "I want a new brother."

Looking at the two of them together, you might not notice the differences. Both are handsome little fellas, very active, always smiling. But spend more than ten minutes with them, and it becomes obvious. Yes, Nick smiles virtually all of his waking hours. He is one of the happiest people you will ever meet. So what's the problem?

As parents, we always want more for our children. We want to know why they are happy. We want them to experience life and all of its emotions. It sounds crazy, but looking at Nick every day makes me wish he would be sad sometimes, or cry, or be afraid of monsters under his bed. Unfortunately, understanding what is going on in his head and his heart is left to speculation. We are fighting a ghost.

Throughout his five years, he has made great progress—so says his Individualized Education Program. Progress, like most things, is measured in relative terms. When measured in each moment, each hour, each day, the pace of development seems excruciatingly slow. For example, one morning Nick had begun to get himself dressed. Like most five-year-olds, he sometimes drifted off and didn't pay attention to what he was doing. He had taken off all his dirty clothes, and we had lined up his clean ones on his bed. For the next few minutes, which seemed like hours, I watched as he tried to put on his underwear. First there were the blank stares at the ceiling, the underwear twirling through his fingers like a bayonet. Then he attempted to put them on, both legs in one side, then backwards. I kept trying to tell myself that the time spent on discovery is worth the investment; leave him alone, and he would figure it out.

Then Joseph appeared: "Dad, I'm all done. I finished first. Nick is still not dressed?" One of the many challenges of twins is we have a constant reminder of how far behind Nick is.

Finally, the underwear was on—but backwards. I had spent all my patience, and then I intervened, fixing them. I took a deep breath, and together we put on the rest of his clothes.

During our early parenting years, Jeannie got her hands on a great book: *Love and Logic: Magic for Early Childhood* by Jim Fay and Charles Fay, PhD. Within the pages, the authors, father and son, discuss the importance of "withdrawals": We spend so much of our time investing in our children. These deposits accumulate and display themselves through our child's accomplishments, facial expressions, and exclamations such as, "I did it!" Occasionally, we need to take a withdrawal. It could mean the intervening mentioned above; it could mean walking away for a few minutes instead of saying or doing something you might regret. For Jeannie and I, it often means confessions at nine-thirty at night on the couch over a Grey Goose martini. We recap our day, confess our shortcomings—as defined by ourselves—support each other, and look forward to another day of opportunity.

Chapter Sixteen

Sometimes I wonder what Nick dreams about. Are his dreams limited to his cognitive experiences, or does he enter another dimension, as we all sometimes do, when he drifts off at night? It's the same thought I have when I look into his eyes. His world seems so simple, so vanilla. His likes and dislikes are clearly defined and rarely change. Introducing him to new experiences of any sensation are very challenging, although a common mistake is to assume his sensory issues are always about what seems visible. When he uses his index fingers to close his ears, most people assume the noise is too much. But really, it's sensory overload. The combination of senses causes him to shut down and take flight.

Through his sensory integration therapy, he has made progress. Take the dinner table as an example: Early on, "taking flight" translated into a mad dash from the table as soon as the food appeared. Over time, this has morphed into a slow crawl out of his seat and now more of a meander to another room for some sensory cleansing. Although it is rare to have him sit in his chair for the entire dinner, he often returns to collect his plate and finds a sensory-safe place to get his sustenance.

Back to dreams: One night, like many others, Nick was awake before the crows. It must have been about three o'clock. Rather than crying in the night that monsters were under his bed or sitting up recalling a bad dream, he was laughing hysterically and clapping. It was an example of a time when I wished he could be something other than happy. Try to explain to him that his brother was sleeping and he should be quiet; or that Mommy and Daddy were tired and needed to get some sleep so we could take care of all his needs in the morning; or that it's night time and he should have been sleeping. The first thing to note about communicating with Nick is that words don't work. Pictures do. The second thing is…there is no second.

The laughter and clapping brought me to the brink of insanity. I looked into his eyes and he only wanted one thing: me. But for Nick, a hug or kiss meant stimulation, and I knew where that would send him. More stimulation is the last thing he needs in the middle of the night. So just when my eyes were ready to shut, he jammed his chin into my forehead. He was seeking affection, stimulation, and I wanted to scream.

I got him to lie down and covered him up. I sat in the reading chair and hoped he would fall asleep and his brother wouldn't wake up. As I drifted off, I suddenly was awakened by a tug at my leg.

"Daddy, I'm thirsty."

With my eyes still half shut, I told Joseph to get a cup from the bathroom and help himself.

I still felt his presence. As I began to open my eyes, I heard him say, "Daddy, can you get it for me? Joseph is still sleeping, and I don't want to wake him up."

As I began to regain full consciousness, I flashed back to the first four months of their miraculous lives: feedings, diaper changes, cleanups, and laundry around the clock. Jeannie and I kept a notebook of Baby A and Baby B so we could remember when the last maintenance was. "At 1:20 a.m. Baby A ate four ounces of milk, did a number one and number two, then spit up most of his milk. At 2:10 Baby B woke, did not eat, did number one…"

I suddenly felt that same feeling of weightlessness, straddling the boundary of sleep and awake: "Daddy, I have been asleep for a long time. I felt kind of like a stuffed animal. People would talk to me, but I wouldn't talk back. They used pictures to help me pick what I wanted and taught me how to sign. Maybe they thought I was deaf. I could hear them, understand them, but I couldn't talk to them. I knew what I wanted to say, but it got lost somewhere in my body between my head and my mouth."

I was speechless. I looked into his eyes, and I saw an awakening. They were as bright and beautifully brown as always, just like his mother's. But there was a difference: a clarity, a focus, a purpose—the look I have felt inside me my whole life. I always knew what I wanted. Sometimes I took stupid detours, but I always wound up where I intended. I have an ability to visualize the preparation, the delivery, and the outcome, and finally the pieces have all come together for Nick.

After a few blinks, the vision before me became much clearer. I was indeed awake, and Nick had his hand on my knee. In his hands he did not have his Elmo or a cup of water, but a message for me. The strip from his Picture Exchange Book[1]:

---

[1] The Picture Communication Symbols © 1981-2009 by Mayer-Johnson LLC. All Rights Reserved Worldwide. Used with permission. Boardmaker™ is a trademark of Mayer-Johnson LLC. DynaVox Mayer-Johnson, 2100 Wharton Street, Suite 400, Pittsburgh, PA 15203. Phone: 800-588-4548. Fax: 866-585-6260. Email: mayer-johnson.usa@mayer-johnson.com. Web site: www.mayer-johnson.com.

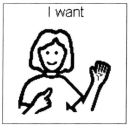
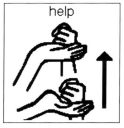
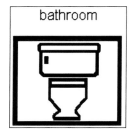

I have had this dream many times, with minor variations.

Perspective is essential in life, especially when you live moment-to-moment. Perspective can be the difference between sanity and a leap off the roof. So taking the glass-is-half-full approach, I still hold out hope that Nick will awaken. He will learn to visualize and communicate his thoughts, his hopes, and his dreams. He will be more than just a happy boy. He will grow into a receptive, responsive man connected with the world.

For now, we need to be realistic about his world. One of the traps was to mourn for the world he does not experience, the sights and sounds, the highs and lows of varied childhood emotions: blowing out candles on a birthday cake, making a list to send to Santa Claus, waiting for the Easter Bunny to come while you are sleeping. Nick is happy in his world, and we need to keep reminding ourselves that it's okay. He is not saddened by birthdays or Christmases past or by kids who don't play nicely on the playground. He simply lives in the moment, is comforted by his familiarity, and loves his mama.

Oh, how he loves his mama. When they embrace, I see many things. I see the deluge of love they have for each other expressed in different ways. Nick smiles and reaches out to her; his body language tells all. Jeannie embraces him with the ferocity of a lioness protecting her cub. Often in her eyes I see her passion to protect Baby B from the demon that has possessed him, that has stolen our boy and not allowed a part of him to materialize.

In these moments, you can see the bittersweet side of Nick's life, the blessing of his temperament, his happy-go-lucky approach to each day. The flipside is that he is living on the fringe; his experiences seem superficial. As he ages, it becomes more difficult to digest. It's okay for a five-year-old to have nothing but love in his heart and to want affection, immediate stimulation, and the fulfillment of his basic needs. But what about when he grows older, when it's not so cute to laugh and clap at inopportune moments? I guess we will deal with that when it comes. Better yet, that's why we have a plan. That's why we get so involved in his development. Keeping perspective means we keep pushing forward and always remain grounded by understanding his universe, not ours—they are worlds apart. Our mission is to expand his world, to introduce him to new experiences, and to hope that the bandwidth of our connection continues to grow.

Nick keeps teaching us how to live.

Chapter Seventeen

So what do we hope for each day? Like many obstacles, we break each day into pieces, taking one stage at a time:

1) We hope he gets a good night's sleep. Much of Nick's day is physical, and without proper rest, he may not attend to his many scheduled and unscheduled activities, which include his speech and language therapy, his occupational therapy, and sensory integration therapy.

2) A smiling face when he opens his eyes. Nick has spoiled us with his electric smile. He is extra yummy when he wakes up. This is probably his most affectionate time, although he is loving most of his waking hours. He wakes up slowly, unlike his maniacal brother who needs about two minutes to turn into the Energizer Bunny.

3) Sustenance: Balance is the key in this area. Nick is quite particular about food. His sensitivities include color, texture, and smell. While we would strive to have him peel his own banana, or even use a fork to help develop his fine motor skills, we often feed him.

4) Bathroom: A good day includes no accidents. A better day would involve Nick coming to us, pointing, and leading us to help him. An even better day would include using his pictures. In a perfect day, still being realistic about incremental progress, Nick would head to the bathroom himself and take care of business. I blissfully would trade cleaning up a straight stream across the floor for some independent actions.

And what about his brother?

Joseph has the acuity of his parents. One of the many threads Jeannie and I share is our attention to detail. Although five years with twins has caused us to adjust our priorities, we both vehemently hold on to many characteristics that we are beginning to see in Joseph. He can remember his bowling scores from two years ago.

Last year we took a family trip to Disney World. While we were there, we celebrated his papa's birthday. He recalls what he had for breakfast (I think it was waffles in the shape of Mickey Mouse), which characters sat down with us, and how many candles Papa had on his birthday cupcake. Was it Chip or Dale who helped Papa blow them out? Joseph remembers.

When his kindergarten class was preparing for the graduation play, the theme was the alphabet, and each child had been given a letter and several lines to memorize. They also would be singing seven different songs. Within the first week, Joseph had all seven songs memorized, had introduced body language to his already memorized lines, and could recite which letter was assigned to each of his twenty-five classmates. For most of the kids, he knew their full names and even their addresses.

Like many of life's great challenges, autism will push you to learn how strong you are. I have mentioned many times that perspective remains the most important element in dealing with this horrible disease. We need to find the delicate balance between hope and reality, never stop trying to understand Nick's challenges, but also push the envelope and reach high. You never know when an unexpected surprise will arrive.

To exemplify, let's take a snapshot of Nick's preschool—not his special education class where his peers included children with similar challenges, but his preschool, where he spent half his day integrated with typically developing kids his own age.

One of our greatest fears was the way other children would react to Nicholas: the fact that he doesn't speak; his hyper- and hypo-sensitivities, including smacking his palm to his chin, placing his fingers in his ears when he is over-stimulated, and his often-unanticipated loud clapping and yelling. We remembered our own childhood classrooms and wondered how they would work for a child like Nick. How would the teachers and administrators be equipped to handle his unique needs? What would be the reaction of the parents of his classmates?

Nick's caregivers have been more than we could ask for, true angels on earth with PhDs in parenting, nurturing, and child development. His classmates have been truly remarkable—an incredible surprise. I never will again underestimate the abilities of a child. I cannot count one instance in the past three years when Nicholas has been treated as anything other than a boy in the class who is just a little bit different.

Nick often is invited to birthday parties, which we dread. Unless the event is in a playground or another venue where he can roam free, it just won't work. He can't sit at a table in someone's house and sing "Happy Birthday"; he doesn't even do this on his own birthday. He won't participate in smashing the piñata or making the party craft. Nick's environment for learning is unique in order to optimize his potential, and these settings simply do not work for him. But one time, one of his remarkable classmates not only made a special point to invite Nick to her party, but she also told her mother they needed to have pictures on the refrigerator so Nick could tell them what he wanted.

If reading that line doesn't give you goose bumps, I don't know what will.

Nick has developed special relationships with two other boys in his class. These fellas insist on high-fives every morning; they seek out Nick to join in their play and are patient and understanding with his unique ways of communicating. Nick has responded by handing them his pictures when he is requesting help. For a child with severe social impairments, this is a major step, and it signifies he has granted them entry into the Nick-Inner-Circle.

So the caregivers have been amazing, and the kids have been equal to the task. What about the other parents? They have been equally incredible. I have seen nothing but smiles when they bump into Nick, which is not difficult to believe since his personality is electric and contagious. There are no funny looks, no whispers under their breath, no pointing. The sad truth is that nearly twenty percent of all children in our public school system have some type of learning disability. Where were all these kids when I was growing up, and where are they now? The short answer is that we don't know. What we do know is that the practice of "inclusion"—that is, integrating atypically developing kids into classrooms with typically developing kids—is a relatively new concept.

We could not have charted a better course for Nick's first few years of schooling. We just have to stay balanced. It is easy to spiral down into self-pity when you realize the reason every parent knows your child. You just have to get out of your own way, put your thoughts and feelings aside, and take a walk in Nick's shoes. He doesn't care why the parents, children, and teachers know who he is—he just loves the fact that they do.

Chapter Eighteen

So how would I describe my son? What have I learned from him?

Those are two questions in which my Dad and Nick wind up in the same conversation in my mind. To some of us, words come easy. To others, they might as well spit into the wind.

At least once a week, I write my father's eulogy. It has been nearly seven years since I delivered the first one of my life, one I thought would come much later—another of life's many ironies. My mother lived a healthy life, took good care of herself, and ovarian cancer took her from us before her sixtieth birthday. When I think back on my childhood, she was my hero. As a single mother, she sacrificed everything for her children. Through the process of discovery, not hard discipline, she taught me the most important lessons of my life. She did not choose to be so strong, so independent, but circumstances forced her down that road. She trusted in me, in my ability to make good decisions, and she is the reason why I am who I am today.

My father is a walking time bomb. If he were a dog, he would be on Animal Planet, a medical miracle. Two ulcers, a stroke, a quadruple bypass, a daily pack of Viceroys for the past fifty years—even after the four bypasses. I knew I should have taken a picture of him after the surgery. He looked like E.T. in the scene when he was all dried up on the side of the road, hanging on to life. Dad was a focused provider, but an absent father and teacher. By choice or chance, he demonstrated how not to do most things: manage relationships, listen, teach, love, and most of all, learn.

So why must we wait for someone to leave us before we realize what they have taught us? Maybe this is why Nick was brought here.

It has been said that the extent of the challenges presented to you are only as difficult as you are capable of handling. It also has been said that out of chaos comes order and opportunity. I would not have chosen autism as the mechanism to see a side of my father I never knew existed, but I am grateful for the result. Granted, having twin boys as grandsons was revealing enough, but the connection my dad has made with Nicholas is truly remarkable.

I always have considered myself a well-balanced person, able to keep an open mind. Nicholas has helped me grow into a person who values and appreciates things in life for what they are, not what they could be. I still have dreams, sometimes big ones. But I have become grounded, humbled, and I train myself to live in the moment.

When I first heard my dad tell my boys he loved them, I didn't long for the reasons he never said it to me. When I saw him change a diaper and realized how proud he was of himself, it was another vicarious moment when his love for my children filled the empty place left by all the things he had not done for me as a child. Seeing him read a story to them provided pure, unadulterated joy, not a longing for what I had missed.

He was always a provider—and that was the extent of his role as a father. Growing up, I always could count on him to deliver life's basic needs. But as I became a father, I realized the varied skill set required for parenting, and all of his shortcomings became even more evident. Today I focus on the love he has for my children—period. I know he loves me, and he doesn't have to say it. I don't have a speck of jealousy for his open emotions, his hugging and kissing, or his pride in telling the world about his special grandchildren. I know he has felt and continues to feel all those things for me. Having been around him my whole life, I developed the ability to read his true feelings without listening to the words. I just look in his eyes, and he tells all.

Both boys have a special relationship with their papa—but Dad and Nick communicate on a unique level. In a strange twist of fate, two individuals who cannot use words to express how they feel connect in a way neither doctors nor scientists can explain. It's not just the jellybeans in his pocket that attracts Nick to his papa. Nick can see into my dad's soul, and he is willing my father to let him, and others, inside—inside a world where no one has ever been; a world where you don't need to be afraid to speak and express what you truly feel, to let the world know you have hopes and fears, that you have regrets for choices you made in life, but you want the chance to make it right. Dad has been presented with this chance. With Nicholas, Dad cannot hide behind the superficiality of his words, as he does with everyone else. The more time he spends with Nick, the more difficult it becomes for him to keep up his defense. You can see it in his body language. Nick wears him down with his hugs, his chins to the forehead, and his electric smile.

One day my dad and I were going through his medical history, joking he is nothing short of a medical miracle to be above ground. I made the comment that he was playing with the house's money, that his break-even point happened long ago, and that, treating his body the way he has, any time left was gravy. Nick happened to be sitting next to us. Dad turned to Nick, looked right into his eyes, and spoke one of the few heartfelt sentences I have ever heard him say: "Nicky, the only thing keeping me alive is that I am waiting for you to talk. After you do that, it's time for me to go."

He said it with a smile on his face, pretending it was in jest. I knew better. He didn't realize he was opening his soul—something he had never done in front of me before.

Nick shrugged him off, put his hands around Papa's ears, and stuck his chin into Papa's forehead. If he could speak, his body language would translate into: "You're not going anywhere, Papa."

Dad melted. Speechless, his eyes began to well up.

Nick's needs are primitive. He gives unconditional love and asks for nothing in return, unless you count hugs, kisses, and the occasional bag of fruit snacks. Nick is pure. He is raw humanity with nothing but organic ingredients wrapped in a freckled, dimpled, milky-white body. His trademark move of placing his index fingers in his ears is symbolic of many things: blocking out the extraneousness of his surroundings, the excessive use of words, the sensory overload brought on by multi-tasking. His response is simply to walk away. Some would call it rude, socially unacceptable. But to learn from Nick, as from anything, you need to sort out the true spirit of the action. Translated into words, his body language would say, "Is this really important?"

Every day Nick teaches us what is important. Some days we get it, and some days we don't. Happiness, laughter, wake, sleep, eat, drink, and laugh some more. Smile, and the world will follow. Nick certainly has developed a long list of parishioners. I have become one of his followers.

One of the many things Nick has taught me is how overrated the spoken word can be. I have spent the majority of my adult life and have achieved the bulk of my successes utilizing my vocabulary. Through the maniacal irony of autism, I have developed a great appreciation for silence, for body language and facial expressions, for staring into the eyes of those you love to understand what is happening between their ears and in their hearts. Like most aspects of this crazy disease, there is no balance.

Can't he just speak a little? We could use both methods to communicate. Perspective remains paramount.

Chapter Nineteen

There are angels among us.

Many years ago, when I thought I had all the answers, a received a book as a gift from a group of co-workers. At the time, I was on the fast track. I had a clear vision of what I wanted, and the way to get it was obvious. To find my heroes, those to whose positions in life I aspired, it was a simple search: Pull out the organizational chart of my company and start from the top, reading the clearly defined titles depicting success. Alternatively, turn on the TV. Who makes the cake? Athletes, musicians, actors—success equals rewards. Life is a process of tangible rewards. How else could success be measured?

I did not realize that wealth makes the quest for self-identity more difficult. I was not born to be a corporate executive; I was born to tell a story, to help redefine what is truly important in life. But although I didn't pay attention to it until much later, I got that book. Open to interpretation, the book is about many things. I later would understand that, to me, it was about individuality. It was about having the courage to question, to be sincere in your thoughts and ideas, and to put them into action. How many of us are ready with a game plan if asked, "What would you do if you ran the zoo?"

For a long time, the gift sat on the shelf collecting dust. I don't think I even attempted to read it, even for the first few years of my children's' lives: one of the many wrong turns I have taken. Thank goodness this crazy world is filled with rotaries. It took me almost forty years to appreciate Dr. Seuss. Watching the Grinch every Christmas only provides a brief glimpse into the genius of this incredible writer. The first lesson I learned is that you cannot breeze through one of his stories. *The Sneetches*? *The Lorax*? *Yertle the Turtle*? They took too long to read. My mouth got tired, and the kids weren't even listening, anyway.

What a dumbass I was!

When I would come home from a long day at work and have very little left in the tank, story time wasn't as pure as it is now. Reading Dr. Seuss is a perfect example. What once seemed repetitive and annoying I now see as works of art and a brilliant method for children to augment their vocabularies. Oh, and if you listen closely (and read the stories twenty or thirty times), you might find some life lessons, too.

Thankfully, I finally got out of my own way and took the time to realize how important reading is to children. As adults, we think we have all the answers. We often act like children when we don't get what we want, and we seem to have lost the ability to understand how a child thinks. As I spend more time with my boys, I feel simultaneously older, wiser, and more youthful and wondrous.

When I finally took the time to read it, it left a lasting impression, so much that it inspired me to write this letter to Nick's preschool, where he spent the first three years of his learning life in preparation for moving on to first grade:

July 18, 2007

Preschool Coordinator
SAU 28
21 Haverhill Road
Windham, NH 03087

Dear Meg,

Jeannie and I have wracked our brains trying to think of a way to thank you and your team for all you have done for our family these past three years. The only way we could express our gratitude was to put it into words.

You not only have helped our son realize his potential, but you have taught us so much about what is truly important. In doing what you do every day, you have touched our lives in a way only few have.

We have attached our feeble attempt at expressing our endless gratitude for the impact you have made on Nicholas, Joseph, and both of us. Please share this with your team of miracle-workers.

(Attachment)

From the brilliance of Dr. Seuss, in If I Ran the Zoo: "If I ran the zoo, said young Gerald McGrew, I'd make a few changes, that's what I'd do…"

This world is blessed with so many angels, yet we choose to most extravagantly reward those who entertain us. The musicians, athletes, actors, and reality-show hosts should be standing in line paying homage to those we need most. Say, "Thank you" to the policemen, the firefighters, the nurses. Let's empty the banks and fill up their purses. And to those miraculous super-humans, the teachers and special aides, let's get down on our knees and pray. These are the true angels on earth. For the reward of their effort is not in their pay, but the smiles they deliver to families each day.

Up to this point in my life, there was only a handful of people who had burned lasting images in my memory: a couple of teachers who challenged me in a way I could not understand at the time, but appreciate now; my first boss, who taught me to be courageous by being myself, and that you could flourish in corporate America by being genuine, honest, and not compromising your values; and most importantly, my mother. I can still feel her sense of concern, love, pride, and hope. Although she left us too early, her spirit lives within me, and I can see it blooming in my children.

Many of life's most challenging experiences have brought me in touch with some truly remarkable caregivers: the oncology physician and infusion team at Dana Farber who cohabitated with my mother's ovarian cancer for nearly four years, and who all wept deeply the day we lost her. I remember my last visit to the tenth floor the day after she died. It was my duty to thank them for their love, nurturing, and most of all, hope. Delivering the news was the second most difficult thing I have ever done; her eulogy was the most challenging.

The NICU nurses who cared for our tiny miracles were also incredible. Throughout the babies' month-long stay, many not only provided the medicine, but also the foundation for what a loving parent should be. They also provided comfort to my wife and me during the most worrisome and confusing time of our lives.

There also were magical spirits who whisked in and out of the NICU, often going unnoticed. Their mission: cuddling. Amazing as it may sound, many of these new gifts of life were not getting enough love. As it was shared to us, volunteers come in to hold, cuddle, and transfer love to newborns whose parents or caregivers do not visit enough. No matter the reason, love is love. Does it matter why the parents can't come, or does it matter why the cuddlers are there? The only thing that matters is that the children are loved. The result? The most powerful force in the universe is provided to a needing recipient.

Maybe it's sheer luck, or maybe you truly reap what you sow. My wife and I take great care in how we treat others, and thus our interactions with angels on earth continue.

When Nick was first diagnosed with autism, one of our many fears was how we would make sure he did not miss out on the opportunity to learn, develop, and grow. We both knew we would be involved in every aspect of his development, but obviously he would need professionals. We just never knew there were so many angels on earth.

Over the years, we have not only grown to listen, trust, and respect you and your Dream Team, but we continually seek your counsel—and you are always more than willing to provide it. Our guess is that many of these angels also have children of their own, in addition to dealing with dozens of kids like Nick who require unique attention and skills and most of all, unconditional love.

Time after time, Nick has made a transition that required changes to his core team: it might be an aide to attend school with him, possibly his sensory or speech coach, his caseworker, or others. We continue to be blown away by the talent, the dedication, the care, and most of all, the results. Progress is often difficult to celebrate when viewed too closely. Keeping perspective is paramount.

A few nights ago, after a long soak in the tub, I was clipping Nick's toenails, recalling how challenging it was to put a pair of shoes on his beautiful feet. We can only guess at the combination of barriers that caused him to turn away anything on his feet: pressure, texture, color, scent. At the time, it seemed as if he would walk barefoot in the snow for the rest of his life. Today, he still puts up a slight fuss when it's time for snow boots. But thanks to our Dream Team, we are a little better equipped to manage the situation, and he is in a much better place from a sensory standpoint.

Nick didn't come with a troubleshooting guide; there are no FAQs for children with autism. Through the help of his Dream Team, we are now able to identify a challenge, patiently work through it, and reap the rewards. Yes, we do get excited that our son does not take off his boots in the snow anymore—thank heaven for tiny miracles.

So now it is time for first grade. But first, we need to reflect on the first stage of the Post-Diagnosis Nick Era. As we embark on yet another frightful journey, we say farewell to the magical caregivers who have touched Nicholas's life the past three years. The team at SAU 28 has left lasting impressions on our son, his parents, and even his twin brother. Just by showing interest in his brother's learning, Joseph has become a (junior) para-professional in sensory integration, speech therapy, and cognitive development. I don't know of too many five-year-olds who can go from watching "SpongeBob SquarePants" to translating his brother's needs through a world of pictures. Joseph knows that when Nick buries his chin into your forehead, it means he loves you, and Joseph responds with a giant, big brother hug and "I love you too, Nick." None of this could have happened without your divine intervention.

As parents, we cannot begin to put into words what the team at SAU has meant to our family. You have been inspirational in creating a clear path to fully developing our sons' capabilities.

So if I ran the zoo, I would grant each of you at SAU 28 a wish. And what is it that you would wish for? A better job? More money? Knowing each of you as we do, I am sure you would all wish for the same thing: a cure. Even though you would be out of a job, I am confident this crazy planet is full of opportunities for angels like you. We need you on every corner of the earth. And anyone who would be lucky enough to have you on their side would be truly blessed, as we have been.

So we say goodbye, for now. Like you, I would have no trouble selecting my wish if a genie were to appear. But since the challenge of autism remains, my secondary wish would be twofold: that families in need will find you, and that they, too, will see you for who you truly are: angels on earth. We are forever in your debt.

Sincerely,
Jeannie and Bill Drover

I have written thousands of pieces of correspondence in my life, mostly to people I have met in business settings. Many of those proposals and thank-you-for-your-business letters helped me achieve success in my career managing customer relationships. Writing that one to Nick's caregivers changed my life.

I guess I shouldn't have been surprised by what was in store for me.

Chapter Twenty

Big job; big house; nice cars; college funds; vacation home we'll never use; lots of income; lots of expenses; kids; a nanny; another kid; stay-at-home spouse and a nanny; travel more; home less; more money; more things; more, more, more.

Why build a family in the first place? The most important gift you can give to your family is staring back at you in the mirror each morning. You can't view it in just any mirror, especially not one in a five-star hotel with a room-service tray outside the door. You can't schedule your children's milestone moments in your Blackberry.

Or, as Dr. Seuss said in *Oh, The Places You'll Go!*:

You can get so confused
That you'll start in to race
Down long wiggled roads at a break-necking pace
And grind on for miles across weirdish wild space
Headed, I fear, toward a most useless place.

And then there are the immortal words of my late father-in-law: "Shit happens."

No matter the reason, the result was that I found myself boxing up my dream job, heading home with a six-month severance package and an opportunity to take a different direction. Since graduating from college with a degree in economics, my focus was clear. I stepped on the accelerator and headed for the fast lane. Nearly twenty years later, my whole world was changing around me. As the band 3 Doors Down sings in "Let Me Be Myself":

I guess I just got lost
being someone else
tried to hide the pain
but nothing ever helped
I left myself behind
somewhere along the way
hoping to come back around and find myself someday.

Since my first job delivering newspapers at age nine, I had developed a strong work ethic. I couldn't remember the last time I was unemployed. Let's see if I can rebuild my teenage resume: paperboy, dishwasher, gas pumper, grocery clerk. My entry-level job at Cerretanni's Supermarkets was carriage boy. I moved my way up to bagger and then onto frozen foods. At age sixteen, I was declared competent enough to do the ordering and stocking of the whole department, while the manager took a nap in the coolness of the milk chest. I guess that's when I became such a connoisseur of ice cream.

From the supermarket I went on to super fast food. In and around Boston, everyone knows Kelly's World Famous Roast Beef Sandwiches. After two years schlepping Howard Johnson's macaroni and cheese and Hood Patchwork ice cream, working at the hippest roast-beef-and-clam shack in the Greater Boston area sounded "awesome," as we would say in Reeveehah! Oh, and working on Revere Beach, chances were good you would also get lots of chicks. Yeah, baby.

During my college years, forty hours a week at Kelly's nearly paid for a semester at Boston College. The hours were long, but the food was good, and the pay was great. I think I actually took a pay cut when I graduated and landed my first corporate job. Say goodbye to my fish-stained t-shirt at Kelly's and hello to a white-collar job in a cubicle.

You can fill in the rest of my resume with some fancy titles and important-sounding accomplishments such as "focused on our firm's value proposition, while at the same time explored new business development." Translation: Our company is good at this. Buy more!

Fast forward twenty years, and there I was. As I headed north on Route 495 towards the Massachusetts/New Hampshire border, I pondered my next move. What do I do now? It should not be difficult to get another job doing the same old, same old. In addition to being one of the medical Meccas of the world, the Greater Boston area also was noted for tremendous opportunities in financial services. But maybe this was one of those watershed moments. (What the hell does that mean, anyway? Sounds good with a suit and tie on, but sounds stupid as I sit here writing in my SpongeBob SquarePants t-shirt and sweatpants.)

It was time for a break, time to be courageous again, to put my family first and reinvest in my greatest asset: the love within our family. Time for the rat race to do without one more rat.

As I scrolled through my Rolodex, I wondered how I would describe my departure to colleagues, clients, and friends. Should I elaborate on the reasons why I decided to move on? Should I discuss my battles with yet another ego-maniacal boss? Not worth it. I kept my composure during the gamesmanship of corporate life. My values were the reason why it was time to leave. I had compromised as much as I could in achieving success.

We all reach a breaking point. No longer did I want to spend all of my emotional energy at work and come home with an empty tank. As I made my goodbye calls, I dug deep into my heart and soul and told everyone the real reason why I was moving on: I had been presented with a once-in-a-lifetime opportunity to spend each and every minute of each and every day with my three great loves in life—not my antique colonial farmhouse, not my black-on-black Mercedes, not even my baseball card collection.

I'm not sure how long it will last, but I am going to enjoy it while it does. I strongly believe one of the reasons I have been successful at my job as an account manager is that my relationships are built on honesty. As I ran through my list of clients, not one of them mentioned an iota about work. Every person I spoke with wished me luck. Many called me courageous for taking such a chance, and quite a few expressed regret that their careers were nearly over, and they had never stopped to smell the roses.

Chapter Twenty-one

Inside is a place where all my Dreams become Realities, and where some of my Realities become Dreams.
—Willy Wonka, *Charlie and the Chocolate Factory*

And so it begins. After twenty years of steadily climbing the corporate ladder, it's halftime of my working lifetime. I need to get out of the fast lane and spend some time in the break-down lane. What should I do first? The honey-do list is as long as the refrigerator door:

- Definitely work out every day.
- We are going to have the best lawn on the block.
- Nooners with Jeannie while the kids are in school.
- By the way, it would be great to get to know the teachers—what a great idea, dumb ass!
- Start writing again: There is a book inside me just waiting to come out. I do come from a long line of storytellers.

Most importantly, I finally get to spend the right amount of time with the people whose opinions matter most. Sounds like a simple plan.

Movie time will be from nine o'clock to eleven o'clock each night, now that I don't have to crawl out of bed at six in the morning and get going. Business travel will center on more important events: the boys' schools, the library, the ball fields. Yesterday, my commute was picking up Cousin Olivia so she could come home and spend some time with the boys.

When I dreamt of winning the lottery, I often imagined what it would be like to have my world be my family. For the majority of my adult life, most of the relationships I formed were through work. Through twenty years and three different companies, I've spent a good portion of my waking hours with total strangers. Over time, these strangers became my friends and confidants. On paper, we shared the same lives: similar educations, work experiences, family situations, and aspirations for success. It's easy to get caught up in world where we all look the same. When you think you have this figured out, test your wisdom by reading *The Sneetches* by Dr. Seuss. By the time you finish your analysis of whether or not you should have a star on your belly, it's often too late. Don't believe old Sylvester McMonkey McBean: We can change.

After a few months, I began to realize why this had happened. It became another turning point in my life, another time to take stock. Being home every day has redefined my hopes and dreams and provided me with the most challenging and rewarding position any man could hope for: to be a loving husband and father—full-time. I get to be there for my family when they need me, not when it is convenient for me and my calendar; to not have to email myself Meeting Reminders for T-ball games and school activities, or to schedule Tasks so I can remember to pick up a card for Mother's Day; to watch my children grow and learn; to spend every moment with the person I met twenty years ago and cannot imagine being without. I have everything I need.

Throughout my various careers, work colleagues would chat: "What would you do if you won the lottery?"

The typical response included, "I'd be bored if I stayed home all the time." Most of the respondents had at least two children.

"My wife would get sick of me if I were around all the time."

"I love my kids, but I would go nuts if I spent every minute with them."

In moments such as these, I felt like a freak. As soon as I got into work, all I could think of was when I could escape back to my family. If I were on a business trip at a five-star hotel, hosting my client at Fenway in the luxury suites, or taking a client out to a fancy dinner, my thoughts always would turn to getting back home. Having practiced my trade for many years, being a relationship manager meant my time with clients was paramount. Knowing where my bread was buttered, I was accomplished at this. Many of the relationships I formed through work were memorable, but they cannot compare to walking in the front door into the waiting arms of my family.

Would I go nuts if I spent all day with my wife and kids? I didn't think so, but I was willing to try it. If I could put up with the corporate bullshit and keep a smile on my face, I think I can handle being around people I actually trust and love to be with. As far as being a full-time parent, I feel the need to experience more highs and lows. For the first five years of their lives, I have seen my kids in the morning, for a few hours at night, and on weekends. That's not enough time to understand their world and to become a positive influence in their development.

Every smart business spends the time to KYC—Know Your Customers. This means not only your children as your customers, but also their other providers. Who delivers "goods and services" to your most precious possessions?

And if being a parent is easy, you are not spending enough time with your children. It's supposed to be hard, even for "typically developing" kids. Those are the relationships that have the greatest reward.

Throughout my career, I have had many titles. Each came with a set of goals and core competencies through which professional progress was measured and rewards delivered. In my most recent position, my title was Senior Relationship Manager—no, not a dating service for senior citizens; my role as account manager would be to get to know my clients so well that their relationship would be deep enough to withstand any service mishaps and still maintain their business. We would put together organizational charts, including all the key decision-makers. The more you knew about each person, the better the connection. Did they have children? Where did they go to school? Where did they work previously? Were they influencers or decision-makers? Countless hours were spent researching the lives of total strangers so I could have one or two conversation pieces for the next meeting. It is a solid business strategy.

Time away from work has helped me reflect on how selfish I have been. What percentage of my waking hours was spent getting to know the people who have the most influence over my life and the life of my family—the people who spend more time with my children than I do? These are the most special people you will every meet, so take the time to get to know them and to appreciate their gifts to the world—and to your children. Tell anyone who will listen that they are true angels on earth.

I see so many parallels with work and home life. While traveling in the fast lane, it's tough to identify the colors of the flowers as you zoom by. When you finally take the time to stop and slow down: Wow! There's that constant state of total amazement again. What the hell have I been doing all my life? I have everything I need right here in front of me; I just need to find a way to make a living at it.

As I reflect back on the thirteen months I spent out of the "workforce" and in my "life-force", I have discovered that I have been given a gift. I got to pull a George Bailey in reverse. Clarence has let me live in the perfect job: Relationship Manager for the three most important people in the world, now four if you include Lizzy, our recent furry addition. I have had the opportunity to meet teachers, parents, and classmates without the pressures of work. I have had the extra brain space to work with my wife on the most important time in our lives, and through it, I have come to many realizations. Most importantly, keep your eyes wide open, for you never know when miracles will happen. And you just might meet an angel or two along the way.

In the immortal words of Dr. Seuss, in *Oh, The Places You'll Go!* (okay, so I really like this book), consider this the next time life presents you with a fork in the road:

You'll get mixed up, of course, As you already know.
You'll get mixed up With many strange birds as you go.
So be sure when you step. Step with care and great tact
And remember that Life's A Great Balancing Act.
Just never forget to be dexterous and deft.
And never mix up your right foot with your left.

Chapter Twenty-two

Ever since I can remember, my performance has been measured and, for the most part, rated high: good grades in school, a bachelor's degree from one of the nation's best colleges, and a successful career.

An enlightening moment happened when I filled out the data-gathering questionnaire for first grade.

Question One: When did your son take his first step?

I could not remember. Was it nine months? Thirteen?

Question Two: When did your son speak his first word?

That was a tough one.

It was as if I was in their lives, but not *in* their lives. I needed to change that. How will this change be measured? Through a development plan, of course. Not sure if my current boss would approve of my less-than-gung-ho attitude, but here it is. Dreaming aloud for my next interview:

Question: So, where do you see yourself in five years?

Answer: I know exactly where I want to be in five years, and for the rest of my life, and putting my fingers on the keyboard is the only means of achieving what I want.

Question: Is there a particular opportunity that interests you?

Answer: Well, I know I don't want any more business cards, fancy titles, travel and expense budgets, or company offsite meetings. And yes, there is one particular opportunity that is of great interest to me.

Question: Can you describe a typical day in your dream job?

Answer: I want to begin my days in my SpongeBob sweatpants, surrounded by the things that matter most to me. Not my big-screen TV, not even my baseball card collection; I want to become a certified expert in my family.

Question: Are there particular training classes you would like to enroll in to further develop your skills?

Answer: Yes. I want to overdose on my wife, my two boys, and my dog. I want to volunteer at school. Why are all the room moms, moms?

Question: How would you define success?

Answer: I want to write a book, pray that some reader will relate and find my musings interesting enough to spend a night's worth of Chinese food on a bound copy of my ordinary life.

Question: I noticed you have been working since you graduated from college. There is only one break in employment over the past twenty years. Can you tell me more about that?

Answer: I took a thirteen-month sabbatical, collected from the government for the first time in my life, and a light came on. Everything became so clear.

Chapter Twenty-three

So that's my plan. Will you hire me?

"I think we are going to need a little more information before we make a decision about your future employment. Tell us more about yourself."

"Well, I like to write."

I don't just write to enable myself to achieve my dream; I write because it is cathartic. It cleanses my soul. It helps me take out the garbage, to unload the burdens I push aside each day, as Jeannie and I strive for a better day and a better life for our family.

Like many other things, life is a results-oriented business. There have been countless days when I wanted to curl up in a ball, get under the covers, and close my eyes. I was hopeful that when I awoke, Nick would be awake, too; that he would be more than a smiling little boy. He would be full of piss and vinegar, side two of the bookend twins who completely exhaust me but make me happy when I go to bed each night. That's what Joseph does: He challenges me in ways no one ever has. Just when I think I've had a full day as a dad, he wants more. But what's wrong with that?

I don't crawl under the covers. Each battle we win makes us stronger for the war against an unknown enemy that has imprisoned our son in a world where the sun shines only occasionally, an enemy that has yet to define the battlefield, leaving us to guess which weapons to use. Does he have diabetes? Give him insulin. Cancer? Chemotherapy. Can't walk? A wheelchair. With autism, we fire shots in the dark, hoping one of them will hit the target: occupational therapy, speech therapy, sensory integration therapy.

So why waste my time writing this? I'm not famous, so no one will care. I have other skills I should focus on. In my various jobs, we would talk about "focusing on your core competencies." I am good at many things, but not great at any. Mostly, I have passion. Once I figure out where I am going, I get passionate and focused and usually achieve good results. At age forty-three, I know exactly where I am going. Regardless of what I do for nine or ten hours a day for a paycheck, I know that my universe begins and ends with my family. If nothing else changes in my life, I still can wake up every day knowing my purpose.

I am married to a woman of whom I cannot get enough. We have spent more than half our lives together, and each year we continue to grow closer. We want the same things, not because of fate, but because we communicate, because we are unselfish, because we make compromises, and mostly because we each put the other's needs first.

Michael Jordan was born to play basketball. What most people likely do not realize is that he worked just as hard, or harder, than everyone else. It wasn't just the God-given talent; it was what he did with it. Similarly, I was born to be a husband and a father. Of all the places my career has taken me, the one I look forward to the most is our home. I have all the challenges and rewards I could ever need within the framework of my family.

Lots of parents talk about how they would be bored if they didn't work. I feel lucky that I know exactly what I want to do, and that's to spend every second of my life with Jeannie and the boys. If that makes me a freak, so what? The fact is, I could care less what everyone else thinks. The only opinions that matter to me are the ones from the three of them.

As an "optimistic realist," I recognize that my dream of being independent, of spending all my days and nights with the three people who were put on this earth for me to love, is a stretch-goal. But what is life without stretch-goals? At what point does a person become complacent and stop reaching for the moon?

For me? Never. Although I have found my lobster, the love of my life, I keep searching for ways to improve, to make her happier, to make her laugh more, and to make her life more fun.

I get my passion and my strength from my experiences and from within. As I think back on the pivotal moments of my life when my character has been challenged, moments when my poise and strength have been pushed to the brink, their cumulative effects has made me stronger. My foundation is from one person: my mother. She taught me so many things through her actions and inactions. Growing up, I had a long leash, and she trusted I would make good decisions. I fed off her strength.

One such moment happened when they wheeled her into the pre-op room, preparing to remove the grapefruit-sized ball of poison inside her. I was tested. In that moment, I dug deep inside myself, trying to reassure her to remain positive. Her response was to return the favor so many infants have granted to their caregivers. The look on her face said embarrassment, as she vomited on herself and on me. But as she looked into my eyes, I felt a strength I never knew I had. My eyes told her not to worry, that I could handle it and much more. I smiled, and I did *not* do what I always did to make her feel better—make her laugh. Instead, I looked at her sternly, confidently, and I nodded my head.

Her response was one of pride. Regardless of the many other choices she made in her life, I could feel she felt pride in the investment she had made in me. I stood strong as they wheeled her off. Moments later, I left the room, my head held high. I felt a great sense of satisfaction that I had the opportunity to reciprocate what she had given me my whole life. For a brief moment, I had taken care of her, and she let me.

By the time I made it down the hall, I was spent. I caved in with emotion, but I didn't want anyone to see me. I didn't want any of her caregivers to see that her son had succumbed to the moment. So I went into an empty room and cried like I had never done before, the type of weeping where your whole body shakes. It was necessary. And in a few moments, it was over. I regrouped and headed off to the waiting room, rock solid—sort of.

Four years and six months later, I would stand before friends and family to express some final words about how she had touched our lives. As I prepared my speech, I recalled that moment of pride in the pre-op room and gathered my inner strength. I knew she was looking down from above, proud that I held my head high and projected my words. I also knew she was laughing. As I stood, poised and calm, I replicated an annoying but humorous trait from my childhood. Standing below the crucifix, in the center of the church, buried behind the podium, my leg was shaking—not from excess energy, as in my youth, but from nervousness. It was an involuntary, symbolic gesture that I see in my son Joseph every night at the dinner table.

Watching TV, eating dinner, playing a board game, the leg-shaking drove my Mom crazy: "Can't you sit still for a minute?"

"No, Mom, I can't. You taught me that."

That's my bio.

Don't be afraid to write yours. And while you're at it, define your dreams.

Chapter Twenty-four

In my dream world, someone will read this story and take a step back. I would hope that such a reader might find my perspective refreshing in a sense that the world we live in—reality TV shows, shock value, upside-down rewards and recognitions—is not the norm, but the exception. There are other freaks out there who get out of bed each morning with a smile on their faces because they get to be around the ones they love, and that's enough. They don't need more.

So someone will read my story and smile. You might also laugh, and probably cry. And in this dream world, I would achieve my goal of financial independence. We'll be on the best-seller list and there will be buzz about making a movie. I have given this some thought and, as of today, Tom Hanks would play me, and for my wife, Diane Lane. Her role in *Under the Tuscan Sun* reminds me so much of my wife: unassuming and beautiful. Not sure about the chemistry between the two, but Hanks is a logical choice for me: simultaneously serious and silly.

The first thing I would do? Well, I would continue to do what I do now, but at a much greater capacity: support the ones who support us. It is criminal that those who spend their days aiding developmentally challenged children barely make a living wage. There is certainly some opportunity to make a difference there. I would contact the folks who run the special education center where Nick spent his first three years of schooling. I would trade a trip to the Gates of St. Peter for handing a giant check to the school administration for a brand-new, state-of-the-art facility. Name it after me, like those who donate billions to hospitals and have a wing in their honor? No way. Name it after you—you angels are the ones who do all the work and deserve all the credit.

So here's my pledge: Buy my book, make me successful, and I will fulfill my promise. Hell, I'll try the lottery as well. Same deal.

That's what I want out of life. That's my overall strategy. Included in my development are specific action steps. Remember, they need to be S.M.A.R.T.: Specific, Measureable, Achievable, Relevant, and, oh shit, I forgot the T. Anyway, you get the picture.

I am so sick of the acronyms from corporate America. We won't have any of those in this new world, except for one: When the recruiters call and tell me about a great opportunity, I will use a favorite acronym from my Sicilian in-laws: W.G.A.F. I will tell them I have a challenge greater than anything they could present to me, and the rewards are much richer than they can imagine. The job is in an industry that is as old as life itself, with employees on every inch of the earth.

The goal is clear, but the path is undefined. Our competition has yet to identify themselves, making it an unfair playing field. We are the only species who will not sacrifice our challenged offspring. Our goal is to nurture them and integrate them into our world. Spread the word, because we need help against this foe.

Chapter Twenty-five

"So who are you, and what do you want with my son?"
According to the National Institute of Mental Health:

Autism is a developmental disability that typically appears during the first three years of life. A result of a neurological disorder that affects the functioning of the brain, autism impacts the normal development of the brain, especially in the areas related to social interaction and communication skills.

The condition traditionally called "autism" is part of a set of five closely related conditions which all share symptoms and fall under the broad diagnostic umbrella of "Pervasive Development Disorders." They each share three primary symptoms: impaired social interaction; impaired communication; and characteristic behavior patterns.

The term "communication" is often misunderstood, both literally and figuratively. Every night, I wish Nick could speak. I want him to tell his mom he loves her, that he is hungry, that he has a headache. Tell her anything. I, too, once fell into the same trap that the oft-visiting family members on the autism periphery did. I took every opportunity to ask his Dream Team, "So when is he going to speak?" I hated their answer, but I am beginning to understand: "First we need to teach him to communicate."

What the hell does that mean? Well, it means that words aren't the only way to communicate. Nick has to learn that he can't just cry or bury his head into a pillow when things don't go his way. There is a continuum of communication skills between "yes" and "no." Here's an example: Nick rolls out of bed and makes his choice for breakfast. He hands me a picture of his favorite treat: fruit snacks. To help him understand, I can't just say "yes" or "no." So I might use a first/then statement: "Nick, first banana, then fruit snacks." In that example, I would recognize and demonstrate many techniques: low and slow in tone. I would squat down to his level, carefully select a calm tone, and use as few words as possible—the fewer the words, the better.

We need to utilize linear communication, to present a beginning and an end. Time is a difficult concept for Nick. I can't say, "Let's wait an hour, and then you can have fruit snacks."

Here's another: Nick is on the computer, and the Web connection shuts down. From downstairs, we can hear him express his frustration. Our inclination is to run upstairs and ask him if he needs help. Once there, we can diagnose the problem and get him back online. We may think we have helped him, but we have failed him. As hard as it may seem, we need to wait for him to seek us out for help. This could be accomplished through a sentence strip from his picture book[2]:

I want	help	computer
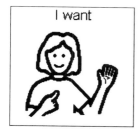	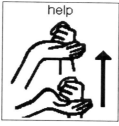	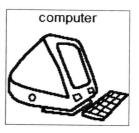

It also could be accomplished through sign language, as Nick has picked up some words, though so far, we have not spent significant time developing sign language with him. Admittedly, it is a white flag to the non-verbal demon that has possessed him. So we augment his visual learning with a few signs.

His primary mode of communication is through pictures. This may take many forms. Nick performs best when presented with a visual schedule. For example: "It's time to get ready for bed." Joseph knows what's next. He often will vary the order of brushing his teeth, washing his face (if you can call it that), and putting on his pjs.

Nick responds best to a picture sequence[3]:

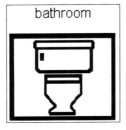

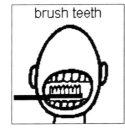

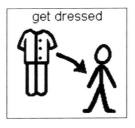

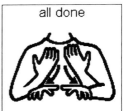

Upon the completion of each task, we remove it from the board or Velcro strip and place it in the "All Done" box, labeled as such.

Once he has become familiar with the visuals, we make the pictures more personal. Jeannie has a library of hundreds of photos taken of Nick and Joe performing various tasks, such as those above. They might also include playing on the swing set, going for a ride in the car, taking a bath, and so on.

More from the experts at the National Institute of Mental Health:

People with autism can be a little autistic or very autistic. Thus, it is possible to be bright, verbal, and autistic, as well as mentally retarded, non-verbal, and autistic. A disorder that includes such a broad range of symptoms is called a spectrum disorder, hence the term "autism spectrum disorder."

Individuals with autism interact with others differently. They often appear to live a life of isolation, have difficulty understanding and expressing emotion, and may express attachment in a different manner. Approximately forty percent of individuals with autism do not speak. Others exhibit echolalia, a parrot-like repeating of what has been said to them. Persons with autism often have difficulty understanding the non-verbal aspect of language such as social cues, body language, and vocal qualities such as pitch, tone, and volume.

Individuals with autism typically have difficulty relating to objects and events. A great need for "sameness" often causes them to become upset if objects in their environment or time schedules change. Children with autism may not "play" with toys in the same manner as their peers and may become fixated to specific objects.

Persons with autism may greatly overreact to sensory stimuli that they see, hear, touch, feel, or taste. They also may not react at all to various stimuli from the environment.

Children with autism often have a different rate of development, especially in the areas of communication, social, and cognitive skills. In contrast, motor development—walking and running—may occur at a typical rate. Sometimes skills will appear in children with autism at the expected rate or time and then disappear.

Autism is a lifelong disability that is generally diagnosed before the age of three years old. However, often children are misdiagnosed or not diagnosed until later in life. A basic rule for treating autism: The earlier the intervention, the better. Although great strides are being made, there is no known cause, and no singular effective treatment.

In simpler terms, autism causes kids to experience the world differently from the way most other kids do. It's hard for kids with autism to talk with other people and express themselves using words. Kids who have autism usually keep to themselves, and many can't communicate without special help.

They also may react to what's going on around them in unusual ways. Normal sounds may really bother someone with autism, so much that the person covers his or her ears. Being touched, even in a gentle way, may feel uncomfortable.

Kids with autism often can't make connections that other kids make easily. For example, when someone smiles, you know the smiling person is happy or being friendly. But a kid with autism may have trouble connecting that smile with the person's happy feelings. A kid who has autism also has trouble linking words to their meanings. Imagine trying to understand what your mom is saying if you didn't know what her words really mean. It is doubly frustrating, then, if a kid can't come up with the right words to express his or her own thoughts in return.

Autism causes kids to act in unusual ways. They might flap their hands, say certain words over and over, have temper tantrums, or play only with one particular toy. Most kids with autism don't like changes in routines. They like to stay on a schedule that is always the same. They also may insist that their toys or other objects be arranged a certain way and get upset if these items are moved or disturbed.

If someone has autism, they have trouble with a very important task: making sense of the world. Every day, your brain interprets the sights, sounds, smells, and other sensations you experience. If your brain couldn't help you understand these things, you would have trouble functioning, talking, going to school, and doing other everyday stuff. Kids can be mildly affected by autism, so that they only have a little trouble in life, or they can be very affected, so they need a lot of help.

If you've seen *Rainman* or a TV show about autism, you may think you know what autism looks like. In fact, though, when you've met one person with autism, you've met just that *one* person with autism. Some people with autism are chatty; others are silent. Many have sensory issues, gastrointestinal problems, sleep difficulties, and other medical problems. Others may have social-communication delays only.

Chapter Twenty-six

As you can imagine, having a child with autism presents many different challenges. It is often difficult to discern the symptoms of his disability from the results of him being a five-year-old boy. Most days Nick is a smiling, happy kid who graciously follows the many requests for his attention throughout his long days. He attends well with his teachers, therapists, and aide. When he is home, we try to remember he is only five, and we search for the delicate balance between continuing the momentum that his Dream Team creates and letting him run free. And like most children, Nick has days when he is obstinate.

Sometimes we think we have his disability under control, and then we get the shit scared out of us.

What's the worst that can happen?

How about standing in the middle of the street with his fingers in his ears? Nick then wandered away. Fortunately, we live in a quiet neighborhood, and a few passersby stopped to notice a cute boy with a red shirt (thankfully his favorite color) heading toward a busy road. So a completely non-verbal child heads off for no particular reason. Maybe he was exploring—who knows? I don't even want to imagine what could have happened. All I know is I shot out of the house like a bullet out of a gun, barefoot, and brought him back home. Thankfully, that phase only lasted a few weeks.

There are moments when we realize that his brother has reached his limit and needs some space.

One of the many cruel ironies with Nick's condition is that he is nonverbal most of the day. Throughout the day, you may hear some babble, some chanting of unrecognizable words, and the occasional "Hi" or "Okay." Like most parents, night time is when our energy level is at its lowest point, and when Nick is at his most awake and most vocal. Still, we attempt tried-and-true methods to help him settle down, to get ready for bed. We have convinced ourselves he still benefits from story time, even though he may clap, cover his ears, and occasionally scream.

As we prepared for bedtime one night, Joseph asked to sleep in a different room. When we asked him why, he said, "So I don't have to listen to all the loud noises." He said it with a slight smile; it was almost as if he felt guilty leaving his brother alone in their room, but was crying out that he needed to break away. So we set him up in the playroom with a sleeping bag, his pillow, and Pooh Bear.

Like most instances when his routine has been broken, Nick was confused. He got out of bed a few times, looking for his brother, possibly thinking it was still playtime. With a non-verbal child, we often are left to guess at his emotions. This can be difficult when he often shares the same facial expressions and body language for many different moods.

As parents, we felt heartbroken and defeated. For the first time since their birth, they had been separated at bedtime. We tried to convince ourselves it was not uncommon for brothers to want their own space. What we could not get past were the reasons why. In that instant, we were reminded that life will not grow easier. As Nick gets older, it will get more and more difficult for others to understand and deal with his condition. There is also a very good chance we will be providing for him for the rest of his life.

Interestingly, within the same day, Nick took another opportunity to take years off our lives. His gymnastics classes have been extremely beneficial in building his upper-body strength and gross motor skills. The classes also have made him more daring; that day I caught him walking along the window sills upstairs in our bedroom. This happened three times. Each time I raised my voice, which we rarely do with either child, but especially not with Nick.

He looked at me, confused as to why I was using this tone. I tried to explain to him why his actions were wrong, but he obviously could not understand—as evidenced by the fact that he did it two more times. The best we could accomplish was to have him shake his head for "No." Brother Joseph would have issued a ticket for a safety violation—his new way of discerning these types of things. Dad just wanted a safety net. This was certainly a challenging moment: balancing teaching with protecting.

Chapter Twenty-seven

Nick sits in the basket, waiting for me. He knows I know what he wants. What he doesn't know is I am trying to avoid him—not because I don't want to spin him around in the clothesbasket and help him get some sensory stimulation, but because I want to encourage him to communicate. We have learned that the act of speaking is not just a physical task involving the tongue and vocal cords. Nick's regimen of visual schedules, picture exchange, and speech output devices are designed to engage him in the act of communication. This needs to occur before he can form words and sentences and sing songs.

So the game goes on. I glance over at him every minute or so. He acknowledges me, stares out into space, twiddles his fingers into the air, and waits. And waits, and waits, and waits. So I write about this challenging event to make me feel less guilty for not providing for my child. Most parents know what their children want before they ask for it. How they deal with it depends upon the situation—with Nick, consistency is key.

After five minutes, here he comes. He points at me and uses his eyes to draw my eyes to the object of desire: the clothesbasket. He leads me over, flashes his electric smile, and sits down. He points at me again. It's a small victory; a more significant one would have been if he had used his picture-exchange book to tell me what he wanted. We spin and spin and spin. His routines are often in groupings of two: two climbs up the ladder on the playground, two slides down the slide, two rounds of hanging on the monkey bars. Once the twos are complete, the tips of the fingers come together—more!

We finally communicate. But before we can further the conversation, here comes his brother with a familiar request:

"Daddy, can you do that to me? Can I have a turn?"

Nick graciously makes way for his brother. He patiently waits for his turn. It's a fifty-fifty chance whether or not he will redirect himself elsewhere or stay and wait it out. Joe and I continue for a while longer, until "all done." They both walk away, off to the next ride in our funhouse.

I can't help but analyze what just happened. I worked for nearly twenty minutes to get Nick engaged, to get him to communicate, and to have some fun. So much of his day is spent in isolation, alone in his room with his books or videos. When he does appear and wants to interact, we try to seize the opportunity. Joseph and I spend lots of time together. He's a sports nut and a math whiz. He loves board games and, most of all, loves to spend time with his mother and father. But he is young, and he doesn't understand when I try to explain: "Joe, you and I spend a lot of time together, and I love being with you. I love Nick, too, and need to spend some time with him."

When this does happen, Joseph will typically nod, say he understands, but walk away with his head down. The crime is that he loves me too much.

Our collective family crime is we fight an unknown enemy that has touched all our lives and that does not fight fair. So in moments like this, I try to regroup, and later I consult with Jeannie about how to achieve better results next time. You could argue these are typical challenges within households of children. The wild card is we have yet to explain to Joe why Nick's needs are special. I wish someone would explain it to us, so we could have a chance at helping Joseph understand.

Chapter Twenty-eight

Nick's constant, electric smile emits positive energy. Being around him makes you feel many things. You feel grateful to be a part of his life, a contributor to his happiness and a recipient of his love and affection. Throughout the course of the day, the roller coaster ride makes many twists and turns, and the deep drops can sneak up on you. In an instant, fatigue can set in, mental exhaustion from dealing with the horror that is autism. Autism moments can turn into autism hours, and often autism days.

Often I feel rage, a rage I want to use against the keeper of my child, this foreign being who has stolen my boy. We are allowed to visit, but we can enter only so far, scratching the surface of his soul. We can see his smiles, feel his hugs, look into his eyes, but we can enter no further. We are not permitted to share in his hopes and dreams, his feelings and emotions, his fears and joys. We have visitation rights, but not full custody of our son.

This cruel punishment is exacerbated by the constant reminder of what Nick could be. His twin displays, often in extremes, the qualities we miss in Baby B. Babble is substituted by extensive vocabulary. Today's torture included Joseph reading the dictionary out loud while I tried to get Nick to stop twirling his underwear and get himself dressed.

Nick rarely cries. When he does, we are left in the dark to diagnose the cause. Nick continuously smiles, claps, and is happy 99.3 percent of the time—but who knows why? That question often dilutes the joy.

These moments happen, and we need to let them happen. In dealing with most of life's difficult challenges, grieving is necessary. In the grand scheme of the days, weeks and months, grieving composes a miniscule amount of our time—but it lingers. We grieve for the loss of a full, complete son. It doesn't mean we love the current version any less, but we mourn for the invaluable pieces that have been taken from us.

Joseph wears his emotions on his sleeve. He has high highs and low lows. Throughout the day, like most of us, he is keenly aware of his surroundings, and he reacts accordingly. Joseph is full of life, vitality, hope and promise. While no parent can predict a child's future, we can see the possibility of greatness in Baby A. Joseph is simultaneously a young boy and an adult man. These moments of paradox happen more frequently, and they bring with them a basket full of emotions. Though he hangs his head when I try to explain why Nick needs special, one-on-one playtime, that reaction is complemented by helping his brother buckle his seat belt. Interrupting our batting practice to make sure Nick isn't standing in the middle of the street with his fingers in his ears is overshadowed by Joseph helping Nick with his homework, often reading to his younger brother, and signing his homework sheet, "Brother Joseph read to Nick tonight."

As both boys continue their physical growth and development, many of the body's processes untouched by autism continue at a typical pace. One day, we all noticed Nick had lost one of his teeth. We had no idea when or how it happened, and we were grateful he did not choke on it while sleeping. I remember the conflicting emotions of that moment. From one perspective, Nick was just like every other kid. He had a hole in the center of his mouth and actually got a kick out of looking at himself in the mirror. From another perspective, there was no excitement about the Tooth Fairy. No time-tested process of parents spinning the yarn about the overnight visit from this magical creature who trades teeth for gifts. Santa, the Easter Bunny, birthday parties—you get the idea. This is a part of Nick that remains unborn: the childish imagination, the wonder of such events that bring sparkles of excitement, occasional fear, but in the end, joy to the children of our world. So we suck it up and smile, and then Baby A steps to the plate.

As we are getting ready for bed, Joseph runs to his room. At first, I think it is yet another stalling effort to avoid bedtime. (He just wants to be with his parents, you dumb ass!) Anyway, he calls me into his room and wants to tell me a secret: "Nick isn't going to get anything from the Tooth Fairy because he doesn't have his tooth. Can you put this under his pillow when he falls asleep?"

Joseph had gone to his secret stash and pulled a dollar bill from his weekly salary of household chores. He isn't thinking about Nick's cognitive ability or Nick's indifference toward money or the Tooth Fairy. He simply is exercising his role as big brother. Once I am able to gain my composure, I realize he would have done the same thing if his brother were "typically developing." Or maybe not. I will never again underestimate how much Joseph understands.

As usual, Jeannie and I consult on how to handle the situation, and we come to the same conclusion. After multiple, giant "I love you; I am so proud of you" hugs for Joseph, we waited until both of them went to sleep. Joseph's gift goes under his brother's pillow. What Joseph does not expect is that the Tooth Fairy makes an additional stop. She also places a monetary donation under big brother's pillow along with a note: *I was watching from above when you gave your own money for your brother's tooth, and I am very proud of you. Here is a present for you, too.*

Chapter Twenty-nine

What's your happiness quotient? Can you accurately measure when you are happy and when you are not? Do you stop and think about why your body is full of piss and vinegar on a given day and full of cement on others? Or do you just go with the flow and let the endorphins pave the way?

By most accounts, seventy-five percent of all communication is nonverbal. Nick makes it clear when he is happy, and it is very often. An optimist would view his demeanor as a reflection of his environment: a loving home, a healthy body, and a world free of worries, blessings every seven-year-old should have. A realist might interject (I have multiple personalities, so I happen to be both an optimist and a realist) that he doesn't have the cares and woes of a typically developing child. He doesn't think about school bullies, mostly because he is protected all day by his one-on-one aide/bodyguard, and his curriculum is one-hundred-percent supervised and monitored. Nick does not understand the concept of time, so he doesn't lament about how many school days are left before the summer comes.

We also have been lucky that Nick has remained healthy. Doctor's visits are a close second to haircuts in terms of a nightmare coming to life. We have tried our best to prepare Nick for these events, but with very little success. One of the practices we have employed is referred to as a "social story". It is an extension of his picture exchange and visual schedules, utilizing visuals to plot out an event. It may look something like this:

Getting My Hair Cut

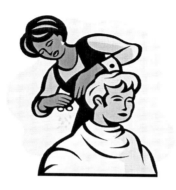

Sit in chair

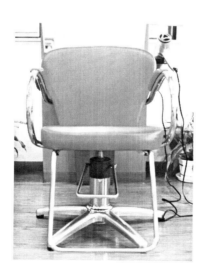

Wear Cape

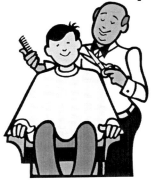

Clippers

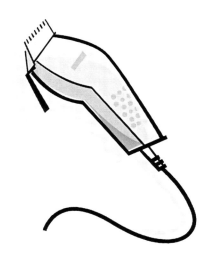

Scissors

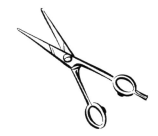

Clean Up

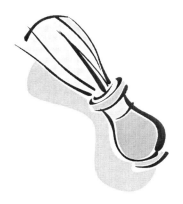

All Done!

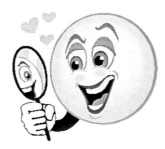

With the completion of each task, we reward Nick with one of his favorite snacks, such as Skittles or Starbursts. The Starbursts work particularly well because the texture allows him to receive sensory stimulation through the rough chewing, redirecting other sensory challenges caused by the haircut. More often than not, Nick will end up on my lap, my arms wrapped around him in a tight squeeze, while the barber works as fast as an ice sculptor in the middle of the summer.

Doctor's visits are particularly challenging. Even though the doctors and nurses do their best, and most have some level of experience dealing with children on the spectrum, the appointments usually are disasters. A win would be getting him to stand on the scale long enough to get his weight. The blood pressure machine, thermometer, and stethoscope are out of the question. Nick will become completely unresponsive and refuse any type of contact, which is rare for his demeanor. We also have been unable to get him to the dentist.

When he was three, Joseph contracted pneumonia and was in the hospital for three long nights. He was a brave little man, dealing with an IV, breathing mask, and constant poking and prodding. If it had been Nicholas, we would have needed to hold him down or have him sedated for the majority of the time. It would have taken ten years off our lives instead of the three Joseph took away.

Joseph has the worries of a typical seven-year-old. At nighttime, he often will dream up fantastic events that cause fear and anxiety. He might ask, "Dad, what happens if you and Mommy die?" Or, "Mom, when I look around my room, I see faces. Is there something in my closet?" And sometimes, "I don't want to go to school, because my friend said he and his buddies were going to beat me up if I don't give them my snack."

Although they are difficult to deal with in the moment, Jeannie and I welcome these opportunities to help Joseph through his adolescence. In these moments, we can see Joseph's gift of performance. We realize not only does he want to stay awake, he also just wants to spend more time with us. It's a compliment, really. In the end, he is bright enough to understand Mom and Dad need to recharge their batteries sans children so we can attack another day. We also realize there are unresolved and unexplainable thoughts and emotions within him that come from being the sibling of a disabled child. When and how they manifest themselves is often difficult to observe and measure.

One of the many frustrating characteristics of autism is the lack of understanding social settings. Nick has an infectious laugh, and his smile could melt a bar of chocolate in your hand. But when he laughs hysterically at inopportune times, it becomes an inner fight to remain sane. Nick's comparable bedtime stalling often involves loud incantations, screams, and laughter. The simple concept of light and darkness provide some structure to sleep time and awake time, but we can see Nick cannot control his senses. When he needs, he seeks. If he wants love or needs to laugh, time, space, and situation do not deter his actions. It's hard to say that there are times when you do not want to hug your son, but when he is sitting on the toilet for the fourth time in the last hour, and you are holding down his pointer, it's not exactly lovey-dovey time.

On the other hand, there are moments when we *want* Nick to show some emotion, to validate his connection with the world around him. One such morning I was taking Nick to school. It was just the two of us, as Nick was attending his summer camp—a nice way of saying that many developmentally challenged kids cannot afford to take three months off, as their progress would take severe steps backwards.

So Joseph stayed home with Jeannie, watching consecutive, taped episodes of "The Price is Right", while Nick and I headed off to school just a few miles down the road. He was hungry and had a cup of Cheerios in his hands. He kept looking into the rearview mirror to see if I was watching him. One of his latest quirks was to use his fingers and teeth to break his snacks into microscopic pieces. It may sound cute, but when you find it in his bed, your bed, the sofa, the empty shower, and the tub, it wears on you. I glanced in the mirror for a split second, and *wham!* My world went spinning into darkness.

When I opened my eyes, I realized we had been hit head-on by another car. Once I hit my reset button, I jumped out of the car, screaming at the other driver. I am normally not a violent person, but I was filled with rage. It quickly went away when I remembered Nicky was in the backseat. He was eerily quiet; not a peep. I climbed over the shattered glass and crumpled metal that was once the driver's side of my car. As I opened the door to the backseat, I was speechless.

Nick was fine. He was more than fine. He remained strapped in his seat. No airbags had deployed, but his Cheerios did, all over his lap. One by one, he went back to his routine of breaking them into small pieces and chewing each one ten to fifteen times. As the police, ambulance, and tow trucks arrived, Nick remained unfazed. In the moment, I wanted to get down on my knees and give thanks that neither one of us was hurt.

When I finally made my way home, I felt a strange set of emotions. My son and I nearly lost our lives in the split-second it took for that oncoming car to smash into us. It would take the better part of a week for me to get my head on straight. Nick's only reaction was a mild fuss when Jeannie came to pick him up with her car and take him to school as my vehicle was towed away. We had broken the routine, as he had to change cars.

That is one of the times when I felt grief for the part of my son that never has been born. I wanted him to be physically okay, but part of me also wanted him to cry, to ask me why someone would do that to us with their car, to explain to him why it was important we both had our seatbelts on, maybe even to have a bad dream about the crash. I wanted him to demonstrate his connection with the outside world. As a parent of a child with autism, that is one of the most difficult concepts to relay, even to the closest of family and friends.

Chapter Thirty

Just smile for me and let the day begin,
You are the sunshine that lights my heart within,
And I'm sure that you're an angel in disguise...
— Jeffrey Osborne, "On the Wings of Love"

Every story needs a hero—or heroine, in this case. Fortunately for me, I didn't need to wait for the turning point for her to emerge. She was there all the time. I guess I should have known it all along, having spent the past twenty years with her. But recently I have discovered that my wife is part of the Angels on Earth club. She is also my hero.

Growing up, like most kids, I thought athletes, musicians, and occasionally the cool family friend (who probably had no real responsibilities) were the heroes of the world. As I have matured, I have come to realize the difference between heroes and entertainers.

The angels on earth previously mentioned within these pages are heroes in the real world. The cleaning lady who worked at St. Elizabeth's Hospital, who probably barely made a living wage, but still found the time to consult and console my wife, often in the wee hours of the morning, is a hero. We don't just remember the keepsakes she presented, but also the blessing of her wisdom, her kindness, and her effort to look beyond her situation and bring joy to someone else.

My wife lay in her bed, recovering from the medications to build the lungs of her preemies—her preemies, who lay awake two floors above her, cooking and growing like baby chicks, goggles protecting their eyes and feeding tubes in their tiny noses. Their lungs were weak, but independent. Try that one on for size, gentlemen: Can you think of a time in your life when you can relate? I can't.

Our angel appeared by Jeannie's bedside, innocently enough. She blended into the scene, going about her business. Through the course of the next four days, she created a lasting impression on my wife, no special deeds and no superpowers required. We all have the ability to do what she did: take interest, listen, console, share wisdom. She is a hero, and like our other angels, she goes primarily unnoticed by the world.

My awe for my wife really began when we decided we wanted to start a family. Over the very long and painful decade that led up to the birth of our boys, Jeannie's strength and perseverance were unmatched. The closest comparison would be my mother's four-year battle with ovarian cancer.

I think about my role in the infertility process. Once a month, I had to go into a quiet room, fill up a cup, and I was done. Occasionally I needed to deliver it in a paper bag if the facility didn't have the secret two-way door located in the jerk-off room. Jeannie's role in the process, which is comparable to her role today as primary caregiver for our boys, was infinitely more extensive. Every aspect of who she was came under scrutiny and examination: mentally, physically, emotionally. The irony of childbirth is that, for nearly a year, women work harder than men would at any job. They typically spend long hours suffering through the excruciating pain of labor and then spend the rest of their lives placing themselves last, behind their children, their spouses, and possibly their dogs. At least, that's what my hero has done.

In my life, I have encountered many intelligent people, experts in their fields who have been rewarded for their proficiency. But our upside-down recognition system is flawed; we have already established that. This manuscript is my attempt to shine some light on the many that do what they do, regardless of where the spotlight is. You may disagree with many of the pedestals I have placed under my angels in this memoir. Where I would hope you would find fault is that there are not *more* of them, and that I was remiss in not identifying all in the long list of unsung heroes.

With age and experience comes wisdom. As I get older, I feel more confident in my ability to evaluate, to filter through the superficiality and zero in on the core, to wash away the dirt and find the gems. To find sense from the nonsense. When I look back on the special people who have touched my life, I see them differently.

Floor ten of the Dana Farber Cancer Institute: the team of infusion specialists, the sales clerk at the boutique, the receptionist—mostly women. Surrounded by the imminent death of their patients, they remained upbeat. If they felt differently on the inside, they did a great job hiding it. When I showed up with my mother to get her treatments, there was a positive feeling across the floor. Yes, I said, "positive". The positive energy created by the people in the room overshadowed the darkness of death that could easily have pervaded the entire floor.

I couldn't see it then, because I was so wrapped up dealing with my Mom, but I see it now. I see it every day in the eyes of the aides at Nick's school, who spend their days working with special children. How drained they must be when they get home, and most have families of their own. How much are we paying these people? Their lifetime income would be a month's salary for a judge on "The Next Top Whatever" on network TV. Their compensation can't be measured in dollars, and most of us will never experience the satisfaction that comes from doing what they do every day. I just wish the balance of power were more equal.

My wife is a member of this elite fighting force. When people ask me about her, I don't know what to say; I don't know where to begin. How can you tell someone you are married to the most beautiful, unselfish, caring person on earth, whose greatest quality is that she continues to strive to do more, to be better? Inside and outside, her actions and her beauty still give me goose bumps. When she crawls into bed with that sexy smile on her face, when someone at school tells me how special she is for all the volunteering she does, when her boys hug her, I feel like the luckiest man on earth. My only hesitancy to putting it on paper is that it might go away. But I do put it down. She is the bounce in my step, every day. She is the reason I get up in the morning. I can't help but love her out loud.

Here's an example of a typical day for my wife: At our boys' school, Jeannie volunteers as a room mom in one class and as a helpful hand in the other. The classes are adjoining, so word gets out when you have a parent who wants to be involved not only in their child's development, but in the development of others. But that's not enough for her; she also wants to make a difference in the lives of those who dedicate themselves to our children. So instead of the typical Christmas gift for the teachers, a gift card or a candle, Jeannie volunteers the gift of time. In her eyes, our teachers give so much of themselves, they rarely have equivalent time for their families. So she creates a menu of dishes for each recipient to choose from and prepares a full meal once the choice is made. This includes wine for the parents, cookies for the children, and a homemade meal from my angel. And the most amazing part is, Jeannie gets incredible enrichment from the teachers "allowing" her to do this for them.

Today one of these meals is scheduled for delivery. Nick's quarterly IEP (Individual Education Program) is also on the calendar. This is a one-to-two-hour discussion with his Dream Team of therapists, aides, and educators on how Nick is progressing toward his goals. Prior to the meeting, we need to shift into a different mode and recognize that any progress is good progress. Forget about the fact that at age seven his cognitive ability is more like that of a three-year-old and that his inability to communicate remains the biggest obstacle; we need to be ready to celebrate that he can touch his nose and hold a pen in his hand.

It's also craft day, so as room mom, Jeannie leads the charge in creating a Valentine's Day project for twenty kids, spending hours of prep time working on a prototype. At the end of the school day, she has fifteen minutes to catch her breath and get the kids settled home from school; Nick typically holds it all day, so he needs help in the bathroom an average of two times in the first ten minutes he is home. Joseph, the chatterbox, fires away at the long list of events in his day, and our speech therapist will be here any minute for Nick's weekly session. Oh, and the dog needs some love and wants to go outside. Welcome home!

Does my wife work? Yes, harder than I ever have in my life, or ever will. Does she get paid? She does, but her compensation is not easily defined. Most of it comes from self-fulfillment. She is special: I know it, and those who spend more than a few hours with her know it, but she doesn't think so. So I guess I'll just have to spend the rest of my life reminding her of how special she is. And how lucky I am. It is a labor of love.

And what will I get in return? The dividends on this investment are currently fifty inches tall and sixty-three pounds in weight. Their balance sheets contain very different statistics. One tells us about every moment of every day of his life. He wants us by his side until his eyes close for the night. His primary mode of communication is verbal. Like his brother, he has an electric smile and gives great hugs.

The other is a little more difficult to figure out. He prefers his solitude and the safety of his routines. He has a small, select group of loves in his life. His stamp of approval is on his chin. When he digs that into you, it's time to join the roundtable. His needs are primitive. He gives unconditional love and wants nothing in return. He is pure humanity, with no preservatives. He is a raw, unadulterated version of all of us, wrapped in a freckle-faced, dimpled smile. If we remove the noise, all the unnecessary layers that muddle up the true purpose in our lives and break down humanity into its simplest pieces, we are left with my son. He is a symbol of what we should strive to be. He takes each day, each hour, each minute as a gift—and that is what he is to us. He doesn't worry about the latest video game, who got voted off the endless array of reality TV shows, or the score of the big game played by grown-up little boys in oversized uniforms. He presents us with life's tradeoffs. Nick sacrifices all of these experiences, which often cloud our lives, and allows us to see the true meaning of our existence: happiness, laughter, wake, sleep, drink, laugh some more. Smile, and the world will reciprocate. We are his students. We are the recipients of his message, and Nick has developed a long list of parishioners.

Like the symbol on the bumper sticker portraying the mystery, he is a puzzle. To know Nick is to analyze each piece and visualize them together. Individually—speech, cognitive ability, fine motor skills, social skills, relation to time and events—they stand little chance of being understood. But like all others on this earth, collectively they result in a very special package, with many layers, some of which have yet to be revealed.

I can't wait to open them.

Appendix:
Information from the National Institute of Mental Health

What Are the Autism Spectrum Disorders?

The autism spectrum disorders are more common in the pediatric population than are some better known disorders such as diabetes, spinal bifida, or Down's syndrome. A recent study of a U.S. metropolitan area estimated that 3.4 of every 1,000 children 3 to10 years old had autism. The earlier the disorder is diagnosed, the sooner the child can be helped through treatment interventions. Pediatricians, family physicians, daycare providers, teachers, and parents may initially dismiss signs of ASD, optimistically thinking the child is just a little slow and will "catch up."

All children with ASD demonstrate deficits in 1) social interaction, 2) verbal and nonverbal communication, and 3) repetitive behaviors or interests. In addition, they will often have unusual responses to sensory experiences, such as certain sounds or the way objects look. Each of these symptoms runs the gamut from mild to severe. They will present in each individual child differently. For instance, a child may have little trouble learning to read, but exhibit extremely poor social interaction. Each child will display communication, social, and behavioral patterns that are individual, but fit into the overall diagnosis of ASD.

Children with ASD do not follow the typical patterns of child development. In some children, hints of future problems may be apparent from birth. In most cases, the problems in communication and social skills become more noticeable as the child lags further behind other children of their age group. Some other children start off well enough. Oftentimes between 12 and 36 months old, the differences in the way they react to people and other unusual behaviors become apparent. Some parents report the change as being sudden, and that their children start to reject people, act strangely, and lose language and social skills they had previously acquired. In other cases, there is a plateau, or leveling, of progress so that the difference between the child with autism and other children the same age becomes more noticeable.

ASD is defined by a certain set of behaviors that can range from the very mild to the severe. The following possible indicators of ASD were identified on the Public Health Training Network Webcast, *Autism Among Us*.

Possible Indicators of Autism Spectrum Disorders

- Does not babble, point, or make meaningful gestures by 1 year of age.
- Does not speak one word by 16 months.
- Does not combine two words by 2 years.
- Does not respond to name.
- Loses language or social skills.

Some Other Indicators

- Poor eye contact.
- Does not seem to know how to play with toys.
- Excessively lines up toys or other objects.
- Is attached to one particular toy or object.
- Doesn't smile.
- At times, seems to be hearing impaired.
- Social symptoms.

Almost from the time they are born, typically developing infants are social beings. Early in life, they gaze at people, turn toward voices, grasp a finger, and even smile.

In contrast, most children with ASD seem to have tremendous difficulty learning to engage in the give-and-take of everyday human interaction. Even in the first few months of life, many do not interact, and they avoid eye contact. They seem indifferent to other people and often seem to prefer being alone. They may resist attention or passively accept hugs and cuddling. Later, they seldom seek comfort or respond to parents' displays of anger or affection in a typical way. Research has suggested that although children with ASD are attached to their parents, their expression of this attachment is unusual and difficult to "read." To parents, it may seem as if their child is not attached at all. Parents who looked forward to the joys of cuddling, teaching, and playing with their child may feel crushed by this lack of the expected and typical attachment behavior.

Children with ASD also are slower in learning to interpret what others are thinking and feeling. Subtle social cues—whether a smile, a wink, or a grimace—may have little meaning. To a child who misses these cues, "come here" always means the same thing, whether the speaker is smiling and extending her arms for a hug or frowning and planting her fists on her hips. Without the ability to interpret gestures and facial expressions, the social world may seem bewildering. To compound the problem, people with ASD have difficulty seeing things from another person's perspective. Most five-year-olds understand that other people have different information, feelings, and goals. A person with ASD may lack such understanding. This inability leaves them unable to predict or understand other people's actions.

Although not universal, it is common for people with ASD also to have difficulty regulating their emotions. This can take the form of "immature" behavior, such as crying in class or verbal outbursts that seem inappropriate to those around them. The individual with ASD might also be disruptive and physically aggressive at times, making social relationships still more difficult. They have a tendency to "lose control," particularly when they're in a strange or overwhelming environment, or when angry and frustrated. They may at times break things, attack others, or hurt themselves. In their frustration, some bang their heads, pull their hair, or bite their arms.

Communication Difficulties

By age three, most children have passed predictable milestones on the path to learning language; one of the earliest is babbling. By the first birthday, a typical toddler says words, turns when he hears his name, points when he wants a toy, and when offered something distasteful, makes it clear that the answer is no.

Some children diagnosed with ASD remain mute throughout their lives. Some infants who later show signs of ASD coo and babble during the first few months of life, but soon stop. Others may be delayed, developing language as late as age 5 to 9. Some children may learn to use communication systems such as pictures or sign language.

Those who do speak often use language in unusual ways. They are unable to combine words into meaningful sentences. Some speak only single words, while others repeat the same phrase over and over. Some ASD children parrot what they hear, a condition called *echolalia*. Although many children with no ASD go through a stage where they repeat what they hear, this normally passes by the time they are three.

Some children, only mildly affected, may exhibit slight delays in language, or even seem to have precocious language and unusually large vocabularies; but they have great difficulty in sustaining a conversation. The "give and take" of normal conversation is hard for them, although they can carry on a monologue on a favorite subject, giving no one else an opportunity to comment. Another difficulty is often the inability to understand body language, tone of voice, or "phrases of speech." They might interpret a sarcastic expression such as "Oh, that's just great," as meaning it really *is* great.

Just as it can be hard to understand what ASD children are saying, their body language is also difficult to understand. Facial expressions, movements, and gestures rarely match what they are saying. Also, their tone of voice fails to reflect their feelings. A high-pitched, sing-song, or flat, robot-like voice is common. Some children with relatively good language skills speak like little adults, failing to pick up on the "kid-speak" that is common in their peers.

Without meaningful gestures or the language to ask for things, people with ASD are at a loss to let others know what they need. As a result, they may simply scream or grab what they want. Until they are taught better ways to express their needs, ASD children do whatever they can to get through to others. As people with ASD grow up, they can become increasingly aware of their difficulties in understanding others and in being understood. As a result, they may become anxious or depressed.

Repetitive Behaviors

Although children with ASD usually appear physically normal and have good muscle control, odd, repetitive motions may set them off from other children. These behaviors might be extreme and highly apparent or subtler. Some children and older individuals spend a lot of time repeatedly flapping their arms or walking on their toes. Some suddenly freeze in position.

As children, they might spend hours lining up their cars and trains in a certain way, rather than using them for pretend play. If someone accidentally moves one of the toys, the child may grow tremendously upset. ASD children need, and demand, absolute consistency in their environment. A slight change in any routine—in meal times, dressing, taking a bath, going to school at a certain time and by the same route—can be extremely disturbing. Perhaps order and sameness lend some stability in a world of confusion.

Repetitive behavior sometimes takes the form of a persistent, intense preoccupation. For example, the child might be obsessed with learning all about vacuum cleaners, train schedules, or lighthouses. Often there is great interest in numbers, symbols, or science topics.

Sensory Problems That May Accompany ASD

When children's perceptions are accurate, they can learn from what they see, feel, or hear. On the other hand, if sensory information is faulty, the child's experiences of the world can be confusing. Many ASD children are highly attuned or even painfully sensitive to certain sounds, textures, tastes, and smells. Some children find the feel of clothes touching their skin almost unbearable. Some sounds—a vacuum cleaner, a ringing telephone, a sudden storm, even the sound of waves lapping the shoreline—will cause these children to cover their ears and scream.

In ASD, the brain seems unable to balance the senses appropriately. Some ASD children are oblivious to extreme cold or pain. An ASD child may fall, break an arm, and not cry at all. Another may bash his head against a wall and not wince, but a light touch may make the child scream with alarm.

Glossary:
Terms I Never Knew Existed
from the National Institute of
Mental Health

ABA. Applied Behavioral Analysis is a system of autism treatment based on behaviorist theories that, simply put, state that behaviors can be taught through a system of rewards and consequences. The Lovaas Institute explains the concept in this way:
- Applied - principles applied to socially significant behavior.
- Behavioral - based on scientific principles of behavior.
- Analysis - progress is measured and interventions modified.

The Lovaas Method of ABA starts with "discrete trials" therapy (sometimes referred to just as "discrete"). A discrete trial consists of a therapist asking a child for a particular behavior (for example, "Johnny, please pick up the spoon."). If the child complies, he is given a "reinforcer" or reward in the form of a tiny food treat, a high five, or any other reward that means something to the child. If the child does not comply, he does not receive the reward, and the trial is repeated.

Autism. Autism is an umbrella term for a wide spectrum of disorders referred to as Pervasive Developmental Disorders (PDD) or Autism Spectrum Disorders (ASD). The terms PDD and ASD can be used interchangeably. They are a group of neurobiological disorders that affect a child's ability to interact, communicate, relate, play, imagine, and learn. These disorders not only affect how the brain develops and works, but also may give rise to immunological, gastrointestinal, and metabolic problems.

Echolalia. Echolalia, sometimes referred to as "movie talk," is the repetition of words, phrases, intonation, or sounds of the speech of others, sometimes taken from movies, but also sometimes taken from other sources, such as favorite books or something someone else has said. Children with ASD often display "movie talk" in the process of learning to talk.

Hyper-responsiveness. Hyper-responsiveness is abnormal sensitivity or over-reactivity to sensory input. This is the state of feeling overwhelmed by what most people would consider common or ordinary stimuli of sound, sight, taste, touch, or smell. Many children with ASD are over-reactive to ordinary sensory input and may exhibit sensory defensiveness, which involves a strong negative response to their overload, such as screaming at the sound of a telephone. Tactile defensiveness is a specific sensory defensiveness, which creates a strong negative response to touch.

Hypo-responsiveness. Hypo-responsiveness is abnormal insensitivity or under-reactivity to sensory input. The brain fails to register incoming stimuli appropriately so the child does not respond to the sensory stimulation. A child may seem deaf, but whose hearing has tested as normal, is under-reactive. A child who is under-reactive to sensory input may have a high tolerance to pain, may be sensory-seeking, craving sensations, and may act aggressively, or clumsily.

IEP. Individualized Education Program. Each public school child who receives special education and related services must have an Individualized Education Program (IEP). Each IEP must be designed for one student and must be a truly *individualized* document. The IEP creates an opportunity for teachers, parents, school administrators, related services personnel, and students (when appropriate) to work together to improve educational results for children with disabilities. The IEP is the cornerstone of a quality education for each child with a disability. To create an effective IEP, parents, teachers, other school staff—and often the student—must come together to look closely at the student's unique needs. These individuals pool knowledge, experience and commitment to design an educational program that will help the student be involved in, and progress through, the general curriculum. The IEP guides the delivery of special education supports and services for the student with a disability. Without a doubt, writing—and implementing—an effective IEP requires teamwork.

Joint Attention. Children seek to share attention with others spontaneously during the first year of life. Joint or shared attention is first accomplished by the caregiver noticing what the infant is looking at and engaging. Infants learn early to seek joint attention spontaneously by shifting gaze between an object of interest and another person and back to the object (also called 3-point gaze), following the gaze or point of others, and using gestures to draw others' attention to objects, either by pointing to it or by a gaze. This desire to share the attention trained on objects builds to sharing enjoyment by looking at others while smiling when enjoying an activity, drawing the attention of others to things that are interesting, and checking to see if others notice an achievement (e.g., after building a tower of blocks, looking up and clapping and smiling to share the achievement).

Ultimately, children learn to talk and use language to share enjoyment, interests, and achievements; and later to share ideas and experiences. Impairment in joint attention is a core deficit of ASD.

PECs. Picture Exchange Cards. A picture exchange communication system (PECS) is a form of augmentative and alternative communication (AAC) that uses pictures instead of words to help children communicate. PECS was designed especially for children with autism who have delays in speech development. When first learning to use PECS, the child is given a set of pictures of favorite foods or toys. When the child wants one of these items, he gives the picture to a communication partner (a parent, therapist, caregiver, or even another child). The communication partner then hands the child the food or toy. This exchange reinforces communication. PECS can also be used to make comments about things seen or heard in the environment. For example, a child might see an airplane overhead and hand a picture of an airplane to his or her parent. As the child begins to understand the usefulness of communication, the hope is that he will then begin to use natural speech.

SIT. Sensory Integration Therapy: Many people with autism are also hypersensitive or under-sensitive to light, noise, and touch. They may be unable to stand the sound of a dishwasher, or, on the other extreme, need to flap and even injure themselves to be fully aware of their bodies. These sensory differences are sometimes called "sensory processing disorder" or "sensory processing dysfunction," and they may be treatable with sensory integration therapy. Sensory integration therapy is essentially a form of occupational therapy, and it is offered by specially trained occupational therapists. It involves specific sensory activities (swinging, bouncing, brushing, and more) intended to help the patient regulate his or her sensory response. The outcome of these activities may be better focus, improved behavior, and even a soothing of anxiety.

SLP. Speech and Language Pathologist. Speech therapy involves much more than simply teaching a child to correctly pronounce words. In fact, a speech therapist working with an autistic child or adult may work on a wide range of skills including: 1) Non-verbal communication. This may include teaching gestural communication, or training with PECS (picture exchange cards), electronic talking devices, and other non-verbal communication tools. 2) Speech pragmatics. It's all well and good to know how to say "good morning." But it's just as important to know when, how, and to whom you should say it. 3) Conversation skills. Knowing how to make statements is not the same thing as carrying on conversations. Speech therapists may work on back-and-forth exchange, sometimes known as "joint attention." 4) Concept skills. A person's ability to state abstract concepts doesn't always reflect their ability to understand them. Autistic people often have a tough time with ideas like "few," "justice," and "liberty." Speech therapists may work on building concept skills.

Stimming. Self-stimulating behaviors or "stimming" are stereotyped or repetitive movements or posturing of the body. They include mannerisms of the hands (such as hand-flapping, finger-twisting or flicking, rubbing, or wringing of the hands), body (such as rocking, swaying, or pacing), and odd posturing of the fingers, hands, or arms. Sometimes they involve objects such as tossing string in the air or twisting pieces of lint. These mannerisms may appear not to have any meaning or function, although they may have significance for the child, such as providing sensory stimulation (also referred to as self-stimulating behavior), communicating to avoid demands or to request a desired object or attention, or soothing when wary or anxious. These repetitive mannerisms are common in children with ASD.

Some of Nick's Favorite "Words"

play in pool	tickle	hug
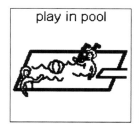	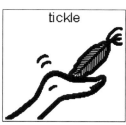	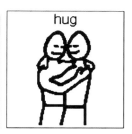
french fries	pretzel	candy
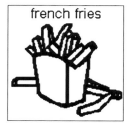	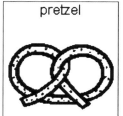	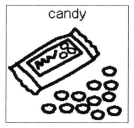
popsicle	milk	juice
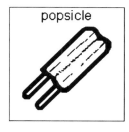	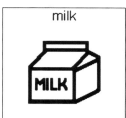	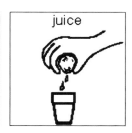

Here's an example of using pictures to get Nick to attend to his Challenger Little League Games: "Let's play T-ball. First put on baseball helmet, then hit ball…" We typically would "incent" him during each phase with a favorite snack, such as Skittles.

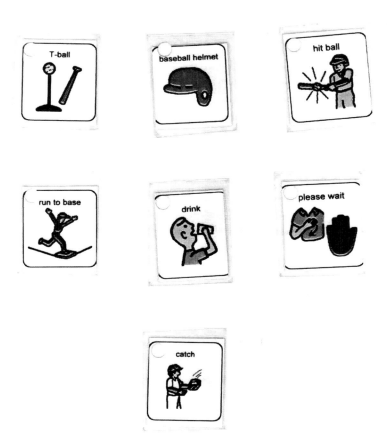